CROSS TRAINING
WOD
COLLECTION

ARIEL WISHERTY

DISCLAIMER

The workouts contained within the 'Cross Training WOD Collection' are intended for individuals who are in good health and physical condition. These workouts can be intense and physically demanding. As with any exercise program, it is recommended that you consult with a healthcare professional or physician before beginning any new exercise program or following any of the workouts in this book.

A healthcare professional or physician can provide you with important safety information regarding your health and ability to participate in these exercises. They can also assess your fitness level and readiness for this type of physical activity.

The author and publisher of this book are not responsible for any injuries or health issues that may result from these workouts. Please be aware that not all exercises are suitable for everyone. If you feel discomfort, pain, dizziness, or your body reacts negatively in any way during your workout, stop immediately and seek medical attention if necessary.

Please use this guide responsibly and listen to your body at all times. Your safety is of utmost importance. Remember, the goal of fitness is to improve your health and well-being, not to endanger it."

CONTENTS

Introduction to CrossFit and Cross Training

Welcome to the exciting world of CrossFit and Cross Training. This book is your comprehensive guide to a variety of workouts designed to enhance your physical capabilities and fitness level. Whether you're a novice dipping your toes into the world of fitness or a seasoned athlete looking for new challenges, this book has something for you.

What is Cross Training?

Cross training involves engaging in different forms of exercise to improve overall performance, prevent injury, and promote balance in physical development. It's a way to ensure that you're not just good at one thing, but well-rounded in your physical capabilities.

In the context of this book, cross training refers to the principle of training using different types of workouts that CrossFit employs, such as rowing, running, weightlifting, and gymnastics. These varied workouts aim to enhance your general physical preparedness, allowing you to be ready for any physical challenge that may come your way.

What is CrossFit?

CrossFit is a high-intensity fitness training methodology that combines elements of cardiovascular exercise, weightlifting, and gymnastics into varied functional movements. It was designed to improve overall fitness and build a body capable of doing any and everything.

In CrossFit, workouts are typically structured as "Workouts of the Day," or WODs. These WODs are different every day, promoting variety and challenging different aspects of fitness, such as strength, endurance, agility, balance, speed, power, and flexibility.

Some of the workouts, known as "The Girls" and "Hero WODs," have become standard benchmarks used by CrossFitters around the world to measure their progress. We'll explore these and many other workouts in the chapters to come.

Why CrossFit and Cross Training?

The beauty of CrossFit and cross training lies in their adaptability and scalability. Whether you're a beginner or an advanced athlete, workouts can be adjusted to your skill level. The goal is not to be the best at one particular exercise but to build a body that's capable of a wide range of physical tasks.

Additionally, the high-intensity nature of CrossFit workouts allows for more efficient training sessions. You don't need to spend hours in the gym to see results. A well-structured CrossFit workout can offer a full-body workout in a fraction of the time.

Finally, the community aspect of CrossFit is a significant draw for many people. CrossFit gyms, known as "boxes," are known for their supportive and community-focused environment. While this book is designed for individuals, many of the workouts can be done in a group setting, adding a fun and competitive element to your training.

In the following chapters, we'll dive into various types of workouts, from classic CrossFit WODs to specific equipment-focused workouts, bodyweight workouts, endurance workouts, and more. Each chapter will provide a selection of workouts for you to try, along with tips on form, technique, and scaling options.

Whether your goal is to improve your performance in a particular sport, enhance your general fitness, or simply enjoy a more active and healthy lifestyle, this book will provide the tools you need to reach those goals. So let's get started on this exciting fitness journey!

OPEN WORKOUTS (2011 - 2024)

Welcome to the chapter dedicated to the CrossFit Open, an integral part of the CrossFit competition season. Since its inception in 2011, the CrossFit Open has become a global phenomenon, bringing together athletes of all levels to test their fitness across a wide range of movements and modalities. Each year, participants from around the world engage in these workouts, striving to push their limits and gauge their progress.

This chapter compiles all the CrossFit Open workouts from their inception to the present day, meticulously detailing each workout with weights provided in both pounds and kilograms. In addition to the workout descriptions, you will find strategic recommendations to help you tackle each challenge effectively.

Whether you are a seasoned CrossFit athlete or new to the sport, this comprehensive collection serves as a valuable resource for understanding the evolution of the CrossFit Open, preparing for upcoming competitions, or simply enhancing your training regimen. Each workout has been crafted to test different aspects of fitness, including strength, endurance, agility, and mental toughness. By engaging with these workouts, you not only join a global community of fitness enthusiasts but also embark on a personal journey of growth and resilience.

2011 Open Workouts

Workout 11.1

Workout:

10-minute AMRAP (As Many Rounds As Possible)

30 Double-Unders
15 Power Snatches (35kg/75lbs for men, 25kg/55lbs for women)

Description:
This workout tests your endurance, coordination, and ability to maintain a consistent pace. Double-unders are a key skill, and the power snatch weight is relatively light, focusing on speed and efficiency.

Recommendations:
Pacing: Start at a steady pace and try to maintain it. Avoid burning out in the first few minutes.
Double-Unders: If you're proficient, aim for unbroken sets. If not, consider breaking them into manageable chunks.
Power Snatches: Use a hook grip to save your grip strength. Perform quick singles or small sets if necessary to avoid fatigue.

Workout 11.2

Workout:

15-minute AMRAP

9 Deadlifts (70kg/155lbs for men, 47.5kg/105lbs for women)
12 Push-Ups
15 Box Jumps (24 inches for men, 20 inches for women)

Description:
This workout is a grind, combining moderate-weight deadlifts, body-weight push-ups, and explosive box jumps. It tests your overall fitness and ability to transition between movements.

Recommendations:
Deadlifts: Maintain proper form to protect your back. Break into sets if needed to avoid muscle fatigue.
Push-Ups: Keep a steady pace. Consider breaking them into smaller sets early to preserve your shoulders.
Box Jumps: Use a rebounding technique if you're comfortable, or step down to save your legs.

Workout 11.3

Workout:

5-minute AMRAP

Squat Clean and Jerk (75kg/165lbs for men, 50kg/110lbs for women)

Description:
A short, intense workout focusing on heavy lifting and endurance. Each rep involves a full squat clean followed by a jerk.

Recommendations:
Pacing: Start with singles to manage the weight. Focus on efficient, clean reps.
Technique: Ensure good form on both the clean and jerk to maximise efficiency and minimise injury risk.

Workout 11.4

Workout:

AMRAP in 10 minutes

60 Bar-Facing Burpees
30 Overhead Squats (55kg/120lbs for men, 38kg/90lbs for women)
10 Muscle-Ups

Description:
This workout combines high-rep bodyweight and heavy lifting, culminating in a challenging gymnastic movement. It tests your endurance, strength, and skill.

Recommendations:
Burpees: Pace yourself, aiming for a consistent, sustainable pace.
Overhead Squats: Break into manageable sets. Focus on stability and control.
Muscle-Ups: If you can do them unbroken, go for it. Otherwise, break into smaller sets to avoid failure.

Workout 11.5

Workout:

20-minute AMRAP

5 Power Cleans (70kg/145lbs for men, 47.5kg/100lbs for women)
10 Toes-to-Bar
15 Wall Balls (9kg/20lbs to 10 feet for men, 6kg/14lbs to 9 feet for women)

Description:
A longer workout that tests your ability to sustain effort over an extended period. It includes moderate-weight lifting, a core exercise, and a cardio-intensive movement.

Recommendations:
Power Cleans: Maintain good form. Consider quick singles or small sets to manage fatigue.
Toes-to-Bar: Break into sets that you can manage consistently without hitting failure.
Wall Balls: Aim for unbroken sets if possible, but don't be afraid to break them up if needed.

Workout 11.6

Workout:

7-minute AMRAP

Thrusters (45kg/100lbs for men, 30kg/65lbs for women)
Chest-to-Bar Pull-Ups

Description:
A classic couplet of thrusters and chest-to-bar pull-ups. It tests your power, endurance, and upper body strength.

Recommendations:
Thrusters: Find a rhythm that you can maintain. Break into smaller sets if necessary.
Pull-Ups: Use a kipping or butterfly technique to save your grip and shoulders. Break into manageable sets.

2012 Open Workouts

Workout 12.1

Workout:

7-minute AMRAP

Burpees (target is 6 inches above reach)

Description:
This workout is a pure test of endurance and mental toughness. The goal is to complete as many burpees as possible within 7 minutes, touching a target 6 inches above your reach with each jump.

Recommendations:
Pacing: Start at a steady pace that you can maintain throughout the workout. Avoid going all out in the beginning.
Form: Use a consistent and efficient technique. Stay low during the jump to minimise fatigue.
Breathing: Focus on controlled breathing to sustain your effort.

Workout 12.2

Workout:

10-minute AMRAP

Snatches

30 reps at 35kg/75lbs for men, 20kg/45lbs for women
30 reps at 61kg/135lbs for men, 30kg/75lbs for women
30 reps at 75kg/165lbs for men, 45kg/100lbs for women
Max reps at 95kg/210lbs for men, 60kg/120lbs for women

Description:
A progressively heavier snatch workout, testing your ability to lift heavier weights as you fatigue.

Recommendations:
Pacing: Move efficiently through the lighter weights to save energy for the heavier lifts.
Technique: Focus on form, especially as the weight increases. Use proper lifting mechanics to avoid injury.
Strategy: If the heavier weights are challenging, plan to attempt fewer reps with good form rather than risking failed lifts.

Workout 12.3

Workout:

18-minute AMRAP

15 Box Jumps (24 inches for men, 20 inches for women)
12 Push Presses (52.5kg/115lbs for men, 35kg/75lbs for women)
9 Toes-to-Bar

Description:

This triplet tests your cardiovascular endurance, upper body strength, and core stability over a longer duration.

Recommendations:

Box Jumps: Use a rebounding technique if you're comfortable, or step down to save your legs.

Push Presses: Break into manageable sets to avoid shoulder fatigue. Use a slight dip to help drive the weight up.

Toes-to-Bar: Maintain a consistent rhythm and break into smaller sets if needed to avoid failure.

Workout 12.4

Workout:

12-minute AMRAP

150 Wall Balls (9kg/20lbs to 10 feet for men, 6kg/14lbs to 9 feet for women)
90 Double-Unders
30 Muscle-Ups

Description:

A challenging workout that starts with a high volume of wall balls, followed by double-unders and muscle-ups.

Recommendations:
Wall Balls: Break into smaller sets with short rest intervals to manage fatigue.
Double-Unders: Aim for unbroken sets if possible. If not, break into manageable sets.
Muscle-Ups: If you're proficient, go for unbroken or small sets. If muscle-ups are challenging, focus on efficient transitions and maintaining form.

Workout 12.5

Workout:

AMRAP in 7 minutes

Thrusters (45kg/100lbs for men, 30kg/65lbs for women)
Chest-to-Bar Pull-Ups

Round 1: 3 reps each
Round 2: 6 reps each
Round 3: 9 reps each
Continue adding 3 reps per round

Description:
This workout combines thrusters and chest-to-bar pull-ups in increasing rep schemes, testing your ability to handle both movements under fatigue.

Recommendations:
Thrusters: Find a rhythm that you can maintain. Break into manageable sets to avoid burning out.
Pull-Ups: Use a kipping or butterfly technique to save your grip and

shoulders. Break into smaller sets early if needed to avoid failure.

Pacing: Start at a steady pace and aim to maintain it as the reps increase.

2013 Open Workouts

Workout 13.1

Workout:

17-minute AMRAP

40 Burpees

30 Snatches (35kg/75lbs for men, 20kg/45lbs for women)

30 Burpees

30 Snatches (61kg/135lbs for men, 34kg/75lbs for women)

20 Burpees

30 Snatches (75kg/165lbs for men, 45kg/100lbs for women)

10 Burpees

Max Snatches (95kg/210lbs for men, 61kg/120lbs for women)

Description:

This workout is a combination of high-rep burpees and progressively heavier snatches. It tests your endurance, strength, and ability to lift under fatigue.

Recommendations:

Burpees: Maintain a steady pace. Use efficient movement patterns to conserve energy.

Snatches: Focus on good form, especially as the weight increases. Use small sets or singles to manage fatigue.

Strategy: Manage your time well. Aim to move quickly through the lighter weights to give yourself time for the heavier lifts.

Workout 13.2

Workout:

10-minute AMRAP

5 Shoulder to Overhead (52.5kg/115lbs for men, 35kg/75lbs for women)
10 Deadlifts (52.5kg/115lbs for men, 35kg/75lbs for women)
15 Box Jumps (24 inches for men, 20 inches for women)

Description:
A fast-paced workout combining shoulder to overhead, deadlifts, and box jumps. It tests your ability to maintain intensity across multiple movements.

Recommendations:
Shoulder to Overhead: Use a push press or push jerk to save your shoulders. Break into smaller sets if needed.
Deadlifts: Maintain proper form to protect your back. Consider breaking into manageable sets.
Box Jumps: Use a rebounding technique if comfortable, or step down to preserve your legs.

Workout 13.3

Workout:

12-minute AMRAP

150 Wall Balls (9kg/20lbs to 10 feet for men, 6kg/14lbs to 9 feet for women)
90 Double-Unders
30 Muscle-Ups

Description:
This workout is a repeat of 12.4, testing your endurance with high-rep wall balls, double-unders, and muscle-ups.

Recommendations:
Wall Balls: Break into smaller sets with short rest intervals to manage fatigue.
Double-Unders: Aim for unbroken sets if possible. If not, break into manageable sets.
Muscle-Ups: If you're proficient, go for unbroken or small sets. If muscle-ups are challenging, focus on efficient transitions and maintaining form.

Workout 13.4

Workout:

7-minute AMRAP

Clean and Jerk (61kg/135lbs for men, 43kg/95lbs for women)
Toes-to-Bar

Round 1: 3 reps each
Round 2: 6 reps each
Round 3: 9 reps each
Continue adding 3 reps per round

Description:

This workout combines clean and jerks with toes-to-bar in increasing rep schemes. It tests your ability to handle both movements under fatigue.

Recommendations:

Clean and Jerks: Use efficient technique and break into smaller sets if needed. Use a hook grip to save your grip.

Toes-to-Bar: Maintain a consistent rhythm and break into smaller sets if necessary.

Pacing: Start at a steady pace and aim to maintain it as the reps increase.

Workout 13.5

Workout:

4-minute AMRAP

15 Thrusters (45kg/100lbs for men, 30kg/65lbs for women)
15 Chest-to-Bar Pull-Ups

Description:

If 90 reps are completed within 4 minutes, time extends to 8 minutes. If 180 reps are completed within 8 minutes, time extends to 12 minutes, and so on.

Recommendations:

Thrusters: Find a rhythm that you can maintain. Break into manageable sets to avoid burning out.

Pull-Ups: Use a kipping or butterfly technique to save your grip and shoulders. Break into smaller sets early if needed to avoid failure.

Strategy: Aim to move quickly but efficiently, focusing on maintaining a steady pace throughout.

2014 Open Workouts

Workout 14.1

Workout:

10-minute AMRAP

30 Double-Unders
15 Power Snatches (35kg/75lbs for men, 25kg/55lbs for women)

Description:
This workout combines double-unders with power snatches, testing your coordination, speed, and stamina.

Recommendations:
Double-Unders: Aim for unbroken sets if proficient. Break into manageable sets if necessary to maintain rhythm.
Power Snatches: Use a hook grip to save your grip. Perform quick singles or small sets to manage fatigue.
Pacing: Start at a steady pace and try to maintain it throughout the workout. Avoid going all out at the start.

Workout 14.2

Workout:

Every 3 minutes for as long as possible complete:

From 0:00-3:00:

2 rounds of 10 Overhead Squats (43kg/95lbs for men, 30kg/65lbs for women)
10 Chest-to-Bar Pull-Ups

From 3:00-6:00:

2 rounds of 12 Overhead Squats (43kg/95lbs for men, 30kg/65lbs for women)
12 Chest-to-Bar Pull-Ups

Continue adding 2 reps to each movement every 3 minutes.

Description:
This workout is a test of strength, skill, and endurance, with increasing rounds and reps every 3 minutes.

Recommendations:
Overhead Squats: Focus on maintaining a stable overhead position. Break into smaller sets if needed.
Chest-to-Bar Pull-Ups: Use a kipping or butterfly technique to save your grip and shoulders. Break into manageable sets.
Pacing: Manage your effort to avoid early burnout. Aim to complete each round with time to spare.

Workout 14.3

Workout:

8-minute AMRAP

Deadlifts and Box Jumps

10 Deadlifts (61kg/135lbs for men, 43kg/95lbs for women)

15 Box Jumps (24 inches for men, 20 inches for women)

15 Deadlifts (84kg/185lbs for men, 61kg/135lbs for women)

15 Box Jumps (24 inches for men, 20 inches for women)

20 Deadlifts (102kg/225lbs for men, 70kg/155lbs for women)

15 Box Jumps (24 inches for men, 20 inches for women)

25 Deadlifts (125kg/275lbs for men, 84kg/185lbs for women)

15 Box Jumps (24 inches for men, 20 inches for women)

30 Deadlifts (143kg/315lbs for men, 102kg/225lbs for women)

15 Box Jumps (24 inches for men, 20 inches for women)

Max Deadlifts (156kg/365lbs for men, 120kg/245lbs for women)

Description:

This workout combines ascending weight deadlifts with box jumps, testing your strength and conditioning.

Recommendations:

Deadlifts: Maintain proper form to protect your back. Break into manageable sets, especially as the weight increases.

Box Jumps: Use a rebounding technique if comfortable, or step down to save your legs.

Pacing: Move efficiently through the lighter weights to save energy for the heavier lifts.

Workout 14.4

Workout:

14-minute AMRAP

60-calorie Row

50 Toes-to-Bar

40 Wall Balls (9kg/20lbs to 10 feet for men, 6kg/14lbs to 9 feet for women)

30 Cleans (61kg/135lbs for men, 43kg/95lbs for women)

20 Muscle-Ups

Description:

A chipper workout that tests your cardiovascular endurance, core strength, and gymnastic skills.

Recommendations:

Row: Pace yourself to avoid early fatigue. Aim for a steady, sustainable effort.

Toes-to-Bar: Break into manageable sets early to avoid burnout.

Wall Balls: Aim for unbroken sets if possible, or break into smaller sets with short rest.

Cleans: Use efficient technique and break into smaller sets if necessary.

Muscle-Ups: If proficient, aim for unbroken or small sets. Focus on maintaining form and efficient transitions.

Workout 14.5

Workout:

For Time:

21-18-15-12-9-6-3 reps of:

Thrusters (43kg/95lbs for men, 30kg/65lbs for women)

Burpees

Description:

This workout is a descending ladder of thrusters and burpees, testing your endurance and mental toughness.

Recommendations:

Thrusters: Find a rhythm and pace that you can maintain. Break into manageable sets to avoid burning out.

Burpees: Maintain a steady pace and use efficient movement patterns.

Pacing: Start at a steady pace and aim to maintain it. Avoid going all out at the beginning.

2015 Open Workouts

Workout 15.1

Workout 15.1:

9-minute AMRAP

15 Toes-to-Bar
10 Deadlifts (52.5kg/115lbs for men, 34kg/75lbs for women)
5 Snatches (52.5kg/115lbs for men, 34kg/75lbs for women)

Workout 15.1a:

1-rep-max Clean and Jerk

6 minutes to establish your max lift

Description:

15.1 combines gymnastics, weightlifting, and cardio in a triplet, while 15.1a tests your maximum strength in the clean and jerk.

Recommendations:

15.1 Pacing: Maintain a steady pace on the toes-to-bar. Break into manageable sets to avoid early fatigue.

Deadlifts and Snatches: Use efficient form and quick singles if necessary.

15.1a Strategy: Plan your attempts. Start with a safe weight and make incremental increases. Allow enough rest between attempts.

Workout 15.2 (Repeat of 14.2)

Workout:

Every 3 minutes for as long as possible complete:

From 0:00-3:00:

2 rounds of 10 Overhead Squats (43kg/95lbs for men, 30kg/65lbs for women)
10 Chest-to-Bar Pull-Ups

From 3:00-6:00:

2 rounds of 12 Overhead Squats (43kg/95lbs for men, 30kg/65lbs for women)
12 Chest-to-Bar Pull-Ups

Continue adding 2 reps to each movement every 3 minutes.

Description:
This workout tests your strength and endurance, with increasing rounds and reps every 3 minutes.

Recommendations:

Overhead Squats: Focus on maintaining a stable overhead position. Break into smaller sets if needed.

Chest-to-Bar Pull-Ups: Use a kipping or butterfly technique to save your grip and shoulders. Break into manageable sets.

Pacing: Manage your effort to avoid early burnout. Aim to complete each round with time to spare.

Workout 15.3

Workout:

14-minute AMRAP

7 Muscle-Ups
50 Wall Balls (9kg/20lbs to 10 feet for men, 6kg/14lbs to 9 feet for women)
100 Double-Unders

Description:

This workout is a test of gymnastic skill, muscular endurance, and cardiovascular fitness.

Recommendations:

Muscle-Ups: If proficient, aim for unbroken or small sets. Focus on maintaining form and efficient transitions.

Wall Balls: Aim for unbroken sets if possible, or break into smaller sets with short rest.

Double-Unders: Aim for unbroken sets if proficient. Break into manageable sets if necessary to maintain rhythm.

Workout 15.4

Workout:

8-minute AMRAP

3 Handstand Push-Ups
3 Cleans (84kg/185lbs for men, 52.5kg/115lbs for women)
6 Handstand Push-Ups
3 Cleans
9 Handstand Push-Ups
3 Cleans

Continue adding 3 reps to the Handstand Push-Ups each round.

Description:
This workout combines heavy lifting with a gymnastic movement, testing your strength and skill under fatigue.

Recommendations:
Handstand Push-Ups: Maintain a tight midline and use efficient kipping if allowed. Break into smaller sets to avoid burnout.
Cleans: Use efficient technique and break into smaller sets if necessary. Use a hook grip to save your grip.
Pacing: Start at a steady pace and aim to maintain it. Avoid going all out at the beginning.

Workout 15.5

Workout:

For Time:

27-21-15-9 reps of:

Row (calories)
Thrusters (43kg/95lbs for men, 30kg/65lbs for women)

Description:
This descending ladder of rowing and thrusters tests your endurance, power, and mental toughness.

Recommendations:
Row: Maintain a strong but steady pace. Avoid going all out at the start to save energy for the thrusters.
Thrusters: Find a rhythm and pace that you can maintain. Break into manageable sets to avoid burning out.
Pacing: Start at a steady pace and aim to maintain it. Avoid going all out at the beginning.

2016 Open Workouts

Workout 16.1

Workout:

20-minute AMRAP

25-ft Overhead Walking Lunge (43kg/95lbs for men, 30kg/65lbs for women)
8 Bar-Facing Burpees
25-ft Overhead Walking Lunge (43kg/95lbs for men, 30kg/65lbs for women)
8 Chest-to-Bar Pull-Ups

Description:

This workout tests your endurance, shoulder stability, and ability to maintain intensity over a long period.

Recommendations:

Overhead Walking Lunge: Focus on a stable overhead position. Keep your core tight and take steady steps.

Bar-Facing Burpees: Maintain a steady pace and use efficient movement patterns.

Chest-to-Bar Pull-Ups: Use a kipping or butterfly technique to save your grip and shoulders. Break into manageable sets early to avoid failure.

Pacing: Start at a steady pace and aim to maintain it throughout the workout. Avoid going all out at the beginning.

Workout 16.2

Workout:

4-minute intervals for as long as possible:

From 0:00-4:00:

25 Toes-to-Bar
50 Double-Unders
15 Squat Cleans (61kg/135lbs for men, 38kg/85lbs for women)

From 4:00-8:00:

25 Toes-to-Bar
50 Double-Unders
13 Squat Cleans (84kg/185lbs for men, 52kg/115lbs for women)

From 8:00-12:00:

25 Toes-to-Bar
50 Double-Unders
11 Squat Cleans (102kg/225lbs for men, 70kg/155lbs for women)

Continue adding 4 minutes and reducing 2 squat cleans each interval until failure.

Description:
This workout combines gymnastics, cardio, and heavy lifting with increasing weight and decreasing reps on the squat cleans.

Recommendations:
Toes-to-Bar: Break into manageable sets early to avoid burnout.
Double-Unders: Aim for unbroken sets if proficient. Break into manageable sets if necessary to maintain rhythm.
Squat Cleans: Use efficient technique and break into smaller sets if necessary. Focus on maintaining good form as the weight increases.
Pacing: Move quickly but efficiently through the early rounds to allow more time for the heavier lifts.

Workout 16.3

Workout:

7-minute AMRAP

10 Power Snatches (34kg/75lbs for men, 25kg/55lbs for women)
3 Bar Muscle-Ups

Description:
A short, intense workout that tests your power and gymnastic skills.

Recommendations:

Power Snatches: Use a hook grip to save your grip. Perform quick singles or small sets to manage fatigue.

Bar Muscle-Ups: If proficient, aim for unbroken sets. Focus on maintaining form and efficient transitions. Break into smaller sets if necessary to avoid failure.

Pacing: Start at a steady pace and aim to maintain it throughout the workout. Avoid going all out at the beginning.

Workout 16.4

Workout:

13-minute AMRAP

55 Deadlifts (102kg/225lbs for men, 70kg/155lbs for women)
55 Wall Balls (9kg/20lbs to 10 feet for men, 6kg/14lbs to 9 feet for women)
55-calorie Row
55 Handstand Push-Ups

Description:
A chipper workout that tests your endurance, strength, and gymnastic ability.

Recommendations:
Deadlifts: Maintain proper form to protect your back. Break into manageable sets early to avoid burnout.

Wall Balls: Aim for unbroken sets if possible, or break into smaller sets with short rest.

Row: Maintain a strong but steady pace. Avoid going all out to save energy for the handstand push-ups.

Handstand Push-Ups: Maintain a tight midline and use efficient kipping if allowed. Break into smaller sets to avoid burnout.

Pacing: Move efficiently through each movement to save energy for the later rounds.

Workout 16.5 (Repeat of 14.5)

Workout:

For Time:

21-18-15-12-9-6-3 reps of:

Thrusters (43kg/95lbs for men, 30kg/65lbs for women)
Bar-Facing Burpees

Description:
A descending ladder of thrusters and burpees that tests your endurance and mental toughness.

Recommendations:
Thrusters: Find a rhythm and pace that you can maintain. Break into manageable sets to avoid burning out.
Bar-Facing Burpees: Maintain a steady pace and use efficient movement patterns.
Pacing: Start at a steady pace and aim to maintain it. Avoid going all out at the beginning.

2017 Open Workouts

Workout 17.1

Workout:

For Time:

10 Dumbbell Snatches (22.5kg/50lbs for men, 15kg/35lbs for women)

15 Burpee Box Jump-Overs (24 inches for men, 20 inches for women)

20 Dumbbell Snatches (22.5kg/50lbs for men, 15kg/35lbs for women)

15 Burpee Box Jump-Overs (24 inches for men, 20 inches for women)

30 Dumbbell Snatches (22.5kg/50lbs for men, 15kg/35lbs for women)

15 Burpee Box Jump-Overs (24 inches for men, 20 inches for women)

40 Dumbbell Snatches (22.5kg/50lbs for men, 15kg/35lbs for women)

15 Burpee Box Jump-Overs (24 inches for men, 20 inches for women)

50 Dumbbell Snatches (22.5kg/50lbs for men, 15kg/35lbs for women)

15 Burpee Box Jump-Overs (24 inches for men, 20 inches for women)

Description:
This workout combines dumbbell snatches and burpee box jump-overs, testing your endurance, strength, and ability to maintain intensity over a long period.

Recommendations:
Dumbbell Snatches: Use a smooth and efficient movement pattern. Switch hands in the air to save time.
Burpee Box Jump-Overs: Maintain a steady pace. Step down from the box if needed to conserve energy.

Pacing: Start at a steady pace and aim to maintain it throughout the workout. Avoid going all out at the beginning.

Workout 17.2

Workout:

12-minute AMRAP

2 Rounds of:

50-ft Dumbbell Walking Lunge (2 x 22.5kg/50lbs for men, 2 x 15kg/35lbs for women)
16 Toes-to-Bar
8 Dumbbell Power Cleans (2 x 22.5kg/50lbs for men, 2 x 15kg/35lbs for women)

Then, 2 Rounds of:

50-ft Dumbbell Walking Lunge (2 x 22.5kg/50lbs for men, 2 x 15kg/35lbs for women)
16 Bar Muscle-Ups
8 Dumbbell Power Cleans (2 x 22.5kg/50lbs for men, 2 x 15kg/35lbs for women)

Description:
This workout combines lunges, gymnastic movements, and weightlifting, testing your strength, skill, and endurance.

Recommendations:
Dumbbell Walking Lunge: Maintain a stable core and take steady steps. Focus on good form.
Toes-to-Bar/Bar Muscle-Ups: Break into manageable sets to avoid

burnout. Use efficient kipping to save energy.

Dumbbell Power Cleans: Use a smooth and efficient movement pattern. Break into smaller sets if necessary.

Pacing: Move efficiently through each movement to save energy for the later rounds.

Workout 17.3

Workout:

8-minute AMRAP (if 3 rounds are completed, time extends to 12 minutes, then 16 minutes, and so on)

6 Chest-to-Bar Pull-Ups

6 Squat Snatches (43kg/95lbs for men, 29.5kg/65lbs for women)

7 Chest-to-Bar Pull-Ups

5 Squat Snatches (61kg/135lbs for men, 43kg/95lbs for women)

8 Chest-to-Bar Pull-Ups

4 Squat Snatches (83kg/185lbs for men, 56.5kg/125lbs for women)

9 Chest-to-Bar Pull-Ups

3 Squat Snatches (102kg/225lbs for men, 70kg/155lbs for women)

10 Chest-to-Bar Pull-Ups

2 Squat Snatches (124.5kg/275lbs for men, 83kg/185lbs for women)

11 Chest-to-Bar Pull-Ups

1 Squat Snatch (143kg/315lbs for men, 93kg/205lbs for women)

Description:

This workout combines increasing weight squat snatches with chest-to-bar pull-ups, testing your strength, skill, and endurance.

Recommendations:

Chest-to-Bar Pull-Ups: Break into manageable sets early to avoid failure. Use efficient kipping or butterfly techniques.

Squat Snatches: Use efficient technique and quick singles if necessary. Focus on good form as the weight increases.

Pacing: Move quickly but efficiently through the early rounds to allow more time for the heavier lifts.

Workout 17.4

Workout (Repeat of 16.4):

13-minute AMRAP

55 Deadlifts (102kg/225lbs for men, 70kg/155lbs for women)
55 Wall Balls (9kg/20lbs to 10 feet for men, 6kg/14lbs to 9 feet for women)
55-calorie Row
55 Handstand Push-Ups

Description:
A chipper workout that tests your endurance, strength, and gymnastic ability.

Recommendations:

Deadlifts: Maintain proper form to protect your back. Break into manageable sets early to avoid burnout.

Wall Balls: Aim for unbroken sets if possible, or break into smaller sets with short rest.

Row: Maintain a strong but steady pace. Avoid going all out to save energy for the handstand push-ups.

Handstand Push-Ups: Maintain a tight midline and use efficient kipping if allowed. Break into smaller sets to avoid burnout.

Pacing: Move efficiently through each movement to save energy for the later rounds.

Workout 17.5

Workout:

For Time:

10 Rounds of:

9 Thrusters (43kg/95lbs for men, 29.5kg/65lbs for women)
35 Double-Unders

Description:
This workout tests your endurance, power, and ability to maintain intensity over multiple rounds.

Recommendations:
Thrusters: Find a rhythm and pace that you can maintain. Break into manageable sets to avoid burning out.
Double-Unders: Aim for unbroken sets if proficient. Break into manageable sets if necessary to maintain rhythm.
Pacing: Start at a steady pace and aim to maintain it. Avoid going all out at the beginning.

2018 Open Workouts

Workout 18.1

Workout:

20-minute AMRAP

8 Toes-to-Bar
10 Dumbbell Hang Clean and Jerks (22.5kg/50lbs for men, 15kg/35lbs for women)
14-calorie Row (men) / 12-calorie Row (women)

Description:
This workout tests your endurance, grip strength, and ability to maintain a steady pace over a long period.

Recommendations:
Toes-to-Bar: Break into manageable sets early to avoid grip fatigue.
Dumbbell Hang Clean and Jerks: Use a smooth and efficient movement pattern. Switch arms every 5 reps to balance the workload.
Row: Maintain a consistent pace that allows you to recover without burning out.
Pacing: Start at a steady pace and aim to maintain it throughout the workout. Avoid going all out at the beginning.

Workout 18.2

Workout 18.2:

For Time:

1-2-3-4-5-6-7-8-9-10 reps of:

Dumbbell Front Squats (22.5kg/50lbs for men, 15kg/35lbs for women)
Bar-Facing Burpees

Workout 18.2a:

1-rep-max Clean

Time cap: 12 minutes total for both parts

Description:
18.2 combines a high-intensity couplet of front squats and burpees with a max effort clean, testing your strength, power, and endurance.

Recommendations:
18.2 Pacing: Move quickly but maintain good form on the squats. Use steady, controlled movements on the burpees to avoid spiking your heart rate too early.
18.2a Strategy: Plan your attempts. Start with a safe weight and make incremental increases. Allow enough rest between attempts to maximise your lifts.

Workout 18.3

Workout:

2 rounds for time (14-minute time cap):

100 Double-Unders
20 Overhead Squats (52.5kg/115lbs for men, 35kg/75lbs for women)
100 Double-Unders
12 Ring Muscle-Ups
100 Double-Unders
20 Dumbbell Snatches (22.5kg/50lbs for men, 15kg/35lbs for women)

100 Double-Unders
12 Bar Muscle-Ups

Description:

A demanding workout that tests your skill, endurance, and ability to transition quickly between movements.

Recommendations:

Double-Unders: Aim for unbroken sets if proficient. Break into manageable sets if necessary to maintain rhythm.

Overhead Squats: Focus on maintaining a stable overhead position. Break into smaller sets if needed.

Muscle-Ups: If proficient, aim for unbroken or small sets. Use efficient kipping to save energy.

Dumbbell Snatches: Use a smooth and efficient movement pattern. Switch arms every rep to balance the workload.

Pacing: Move efficiently through each movement to save energy for the later rounds.

Workout 18.4

Workout:

For Time:

21-15-9 reps of:

Deadlifts (102kg/225lbs for men, 70kg/155lbs for women)
Handstand Push-Ups

21-15-9 reps of:

Deadlifts (143kg/315lbs for men, 93kg/205lbs for women)
50-ft Handstand Walk after each set of 21, 15, 9

Description:
This workout combines heavy deadlifts with gymnastic movements, testing your strength, skill, and ability to handle heavy loads under fatigue.

Recommendations:
Deadlifts: Maintain proper form to protect your back. Break into manageable sets early to avoid burnout.

Handstand Push-Ups: Maintain a tight midline and use efficient kipping if allowed. Break into smaller sets to avoid failure.

Handstand Walks: Focus on maintaining balance and control. Practice efficient transitions.

Pacing: Start at a steady pace and aim to maintain it. Avoid going all out at the beginning.

Workout 18.5 (Repeat of 11.6)

Workout:

7-minute AMRAP

3 Thrusters (43kg/95lbs for men, 29.5kg/65lbs for women)
3 Chest-to-Bar Pull-Ups
6 Thrusters
6 Chest-to-Bar Pull-Ups
9 Thrusters
9 Chest-to-Bar Pull-Ups

Continue adding 3 reps to each movement each round.

Description:
A classic couplet of thrusters and chest-to-bar pull-ups, testing your power, endurance, and ability to handle increasing reps under fatigue.

Recommendations:
Thrusters: Find a rhythm and pace that you can maintain. Break into manageable sets to avoid burning out.
Chest-to-Bar Pull-Ups: Use a kipping or butterfly technique to save your grip and shoulders. Break into smaller sets early to avoid failure.
Pacing: Start at a steady pace and aim to maintain it. Avoid going all out at the beginning.

2019 Open Workouts

Workout 19.1

Workout:

15-minute AMRAP

19 Wall Balls (9kg/20lbs to 10 feet for men, 6kg/14lbs to 9 feet for women)
19-calorie Row

Description:
A straightforward couplet that tests your cardiovascular endurance, leg strength, and ability to maintain a steady pace over a long period.

Recommendations:
Wall Balls: Aim for unbroken sets or break into manageable sets with short rest. Focus on maintaining a smooth, consistent rhythm.

Row: Maintain a steady pace that allows you to recover while still keeping a strong output. Use efficient rowing technique to conserve energy.

Pacing: Start at a sustainable pace and try to keep your rounds consistent throughout the 15 minutes.

Workout 19.2

Workout:

Beginning on an 8-minute clock, complete:

If completed before 8 minutes, add 4 minutes to the clock and proceed:

25 Toes-to-Bar

50 Double-Unders

15 Squat Cleans (61kg/135lbs for men, 43kg/95lbs for women)

25 Toes-to-Bar

50 Double-Unders

13 Squat Cleans (84kg/185lbs for men, 56.5kg/125lbs for women)

Description:

A time-based workout with progressively heavier squat cleans, testing your gymnastics skill, cardiovascular endurance, and lifting capacity.

Recommendations:

Toes-to-Bar: Break into manageable sets early to avoid grip fatigue.

Double-Unders: Aim for unbroken sets if proficient. Break into manageable sets if necessary to maintain rhythm.

Squat Cleans: Use efficient technique and quick singles if necessary. Focus on maintaining good form as the weight increases.

Pacing: Move quickly but efficiently through the early rounds to allow more time for the heavier lifts.

Workout 19.3

Workout:

For Time (10-minute time cap):

200-ft Dumbbell Overhead Lunge (22.5kg/50lbs for men, 15kg/35lbs for women)
50 Dumbbell Box Step-Ups (22.5kg/50lbs for men, 15kg/35lbs for women; 24 inches for men, 20 inches for women)
50 Strict Handstand Push-Ups
200-ft Handstand Walk

Description:
A chipper workout that tests your shoulder stability, leg strength, and gymnastic skill.

Recommendations:
Dumbbell Overhead Lunge: Focus on maintaining a stable overhead position. Take steady steps and keep your core tight.
Dumbbell Box Step-Ups: Maintain a steady pace and switch legs frequently to balance the workload.
Strict Handstand Push-Ups: Break into small sets early to avoid burnout. Maintain a tight midline and efficient technique.
Handstand Walk: Focus on maintaining balance and control. Practice efficient transitions.
Pacing: Move efficiently through each movement to save energy for the later parts of the workout.

Workout 19.4

Workout:

For Time:

3 rounds of:

10 Snatches (43kg/95lbs for men, 29.5kg/65lbs for women)
12 Bar-Facing Burpees

Rest 3 minutes, then:

3 rounds of:

10 bar muscle-ups
12 bar-facing burpees

Description:
A two-part workout with a focus on snatches and burpees in the first part, and bar muscle-ups and burpees in the second part, testing your strength, skill, and endurance.

Recommendations:
Snatches: Use a hook grip and perform quick singles or small sets to manage fatigue. Focus on efficient technique.
Bar-Facing Burpees: Maintain a steady pace and use efficient movement patterns.
Bar Muscle-Ups: If proficient, aim for unbroken or small sets. Use efficient kipping to save energy.
Pacing: Move quickly but efficiently through the first part to maximize your rest time. Maintain a steady pace in the second part.

Workout 19.5

Workout:

For Time:

33-27-21-15-9 reps of:

Thrusters (43kg/95lbs for men, 29.5kg/65lbs for women)
Chest-to-Bar Pull-Ups

Description:

A descending ladder of thrusters and chest-to-bar pull-ups that tests your endurance, power, and ability to maintain intensity over multiple rounds.

Recommendations:

Thrusters: Find a rhythm and pace that you can maintain. Break into manageable sets to avoid burning out.
Chest-to-Bar Pull-Ups: Use a kipping or butterfly technique to save your grip and shoulders. Break into smaller sets early to avoid failure.
Pacing: Start at a steady pace and aim to maintain it. Avoid going all out at the beginning.

2020 Open Workouts

Workout 20.1

Workout:

For Time:

Time cap: 15 minutes

10 rounds of

8 Ground-to-Overheads (43kg/95lbs for men, 29.5kg/65lbs for women)
10 Bar-Facing Burpees

Description:
A couplet of ground-to-overheads and bar-facing burpees, testing your strength, endurance, and ability to maintain a high pace.

Recommendations:
Ground-to-Overheads: Use a clean and jerk or a snatch, whichever you are more efficient with. Break into manageable sets early to avoid burnout.
Bar-Facing Burpees: Maintain a steady, controlled pace. Use efficient movement patterns to conserve energy.
Pacing: Start at a consistent, sustainable pace and aim to maintain it throughout the workout.

Workout 20.2

Workout:

20-minute AMRAP

4 Dumbbell Thrusters (22.5kg/50lbs for men, 15kg/35lbs for women)
6 Toes-to-Bar
24 Double-Unders

Description:
A triplet that tests your strength, gymnastics skill, and cardio capacity.

Recommendations:
Dumbbell Thrusters: Use a smooth and efficient movement pattern. Focus on breathing and staying consistent.
Toes-to-Bar: Break into manageable sets early to avoid grip fatigue.
Double-Unders: Aim for unbroken sets if proficient. Break into manageable sets if necessary to maintain rhythm.
Pacing: Start at a steady pace and aim to maintain it throughout the workout.

Workout 20.3

Workout:

For Time:

Time cap: 9 minutes

21-15-9 reps of:

Deadlifts (102kg/225lbs for men, 70kg/155lbs for women)
Handstand Push-Ups

Then, 21-15-9 reps of:

Deadlifts (143kg/315lbs for men, 93kg/205lbs for women)
Handstand Walks

Description:
A two-part workout with a descending ladder of deadlifts and hand-

stand push-ups followed by a heavier ladder of deadlifts and hand-stand walks, testing your strength, skill, and endurance.

Recommendations:

Deadlifts: Maintain proper form to protect your back. Break into manageable sets early to avoid burnout.

Handstand Push-Ups: Maintain a tight midline and use efficient kipping if allowed. Break into smaller sets to avoid failure.

Handstand Walks: Focus on maintaining balance and control. Practice efficient transitions.

Pacing: Move efficiently through each movement to save energy for the later parts of the workout.

Workout 20.4

Workout:

For Time:

Time cap: 20 minutes

30 Box Jumps (24 inches for men, 20 inches for women)
15 Clean and Jerks (61kg/135lbs for men, 43kg/95lbs for women)
30 Box Jumps
15 Clean and Jerks (83kg/185lbs for men, 61kg/135lbs for women)
30 Box Jumps
10 Clean and Jerks (102kg/225lbs for men, 70kg/155lbs for women)
30 Box Jumps
10 Clean and Jerks (125kg/275lbs for men, 83kg/185lbs for women)

Description:

A workout that combines box jumps with progressively heavier clean and jerks, testing your strength, power, and endurance.

Recommendations:

Box Jumps: Use a steady, controlled pace. Step down from the box if needed to conserve energy.

Clean and Jerks: Use efficient technique and quick singles if necessary. Focus on maintaining good form as the weight increases.

Pacing: Start at a consistent, sustainable pace and aim to maintain it throughout the workout.

Workout 20.5

Workout:

For Time:

Partition any way

Time cap: 20 minutes

40 Ring Muscle-Ups
80-calorie Row
120 Wall Balls (9kg/20lbs to 10 feet for men, 6kg/14lbs to 9 feet for women)

Description:

A workout that allows for partitioning of reps, testing your strategy, muscle endurance, and cardiovascular capacity.

Recommendations:

Strategy: Plan your partitioning strategy based on your strengths and weaknesses. Consider breaking the workout into manageable sets to avoid early fatigue.

Ring Muscle-Ups: If proficient, aim for unbroken or small sets. Use efficient kipping to save energy.

Row: Maintain a consistent pace that allows you to recover while still keeping a strong output.

Wall Balls: Aim for unbroken sets if possible, or break into smaller sets with short rest.

Pacing: Move efficiently through each movement to save energy for the later parts of the workout.

2021 Open Workouts

Workout 21.1

Workout:

For Time:

Time cap: 15 minutes

1 Wall Walk
10 Double-Unders
3 Wall Walks
30 Double-Unders
6 Wall Walks
60 Double-Unders
9 Wall Walks
90 Double-Unders
15 Wall Walks
150 Double-Unders

Description:

A combination of wall walks and double-unders, testing your shoulder stability, coordination, and ability to maintain intensity under fatigue.

Recommendations:

Wall Walks: Focus on maintaining control and using efficient movement patterns. Rest briefly between reps if necessary.

Double-Unders: Aim for unbroken sets if proficient. Break into manageable sets if necessary to maintain rhythm.

Pacing: Start at a consistent, sustainable pace and aim to maintain it throughout the workout.

Workout 21.2 (Repeat of 17.1)

Workout:

For Time:

Time cap: 20 minutes

10 Dumbbell Snatches (22.5kg/50lbs for men, 15kg/35lbs for women)

15 Burpee Box Jump-Overs (24 inches for men, 20 inches for women)

20 Dumbbell Snatches (22.5kg/50lbs for men, 15kg/35lbs for women)

15 Burpee Box Jump-Overs (24 inches for men, 20 inches for women)

30 Dumbbell Snatches (22.5kg/50lbs for men, 15kg/35lbs for women)

15 Burpee Box Jump-Overs (24 inches for men, 20 inches for women)

40 Dumbbell Snatches (22.5kg/50lbs for men, 15kg/35lbs for

women)

15 Burpee Box Jump-Overs (24 inches for men, 20 inches for women)

50 Dumbbell Snatches (22.5kg/50lbs for men, 15kg/35lbs for women)

15 Burpee Box Jump-Overs (24 inches for men, 20 inches for women)

Description:

A couplet of dumbbell snatches and burpee box jump-overs, testing your endurance, strength, and ability to maintain a high pace.

Recommendations:

Dumbbell Snatches: Use a smooth and efficient movement pattern. Switch hands in the air to save time.

Burpee Box Jump-Overs: Maintain a steady, controlled pace. Step down from the box if needed to conserve energy.

Pacing: Start at a steady pace and aim to maintain it throughout the workout.

Workout 21.3

Workout:

For Time:

Time cap: 15 minutes

15 Front Squats (52.5kg/115lbs for men, 35kg/75lbs for women)

30 Toes-to-Bar

15 Thrusters (52.5kg/115lbs for men, 35kg/75lbs for women)

15 Front Squats (61kg/135lbs for men, 43kg/95lbs for women)

30 Chest-to-Bar Pull-Ups

15 Thrusters (61kg/135lbs for men, 43kg/95lbs for women)

15 Front Squats (70kg/155lbs for men, 47.5kg/105lbs for women)
30 Bar Muscle-Ups
15 Thrusters (70kg/155lbs for men, 47.5kg/105lbs for women)

Description:
A combination of front squats, gymnastics, and thrusters, testing your strength, skill, and endurance.

Recommendations:
Front Squats and Thrusters: Focus on maintaining a strong front rack position. Break into manageable sets to avoid early fatigue.
Toes-to-Bar and Chest-to-Bar Pull-Ups: Break into manageable sets early to avoid grip fatigue. Use efficient kipping to save energy.
Bar Muscle-Ups: If proficient, aim for unbroken or small sets. Use efficient kipping to save energy.
Pacing: Move efficiently through each movement to save energy for the later parts of the workout.

Workout 21.4 (Immediately following 21.3)

Workout:

7-minute window to establish a 1-rep-max complex of:

1 Deadlift
1 Clean
1 Hang Clean
1 Jerk

Description:
A strength test following a metabolic workout, testing your ability to lift under fatigue.

Recommendations:
Strategy: Plan your attempts. Start with a safe weight and make incremental increases. Allow enough rest between attempts to maximise your lifts.
Technique: Focus on maintaining good form and efficient movement patterns. Use the hang clean to prepare for a strong jerk.
Pacing: Use the 7 minutes wisely, planning for 2-3 attempts based on how fatigued you feel after 21.3.

2022 Open Workouts

Workout 22.1

Workout:

15-minute AMRAP

3 Wall Walks
12 Dumbbell Snatches (22.5kg/50lbs for men, 15kg/35lbs for women)
15 Box Jump-Overs (24 inches for men, 20 inches for women)

Description:
A triplet that tests your shoulder stability, strength, and cardio capacity with wall walks, dumbbell snatches, and box jump-overs.

Recommendations:
Wall Walks: Maintain control and use efficient movement patterns. Rest briefly between reps if necessary.
Dumbbell Snatches: Use a smooth and efficient movement pattern. Switch hands in the air to save time.

Box Jump-Overs: Use a steady, controlled pace. Consider stepping down from the box to conserve energy.

Pacing: Start at a steady pace and aim to maintain it throughout the workout. Avoid going all out at the beginning.

Workout 22.2

Workout:

For Time:

Time cap: 10 minutes

1-2-3-4-5-6-7-8-9-10-11-12-13-14-15-14-13-12-11-10-9-8-7-6-5-4-3-2-1 reps of:

Deadlifts (102kg/225lbs for men, 70kg/155lbs for women)
Bar-Facing Burpees

Description:
A pyramid workout that tests your strength and cardio capacity with a high volume of deadlifts and bar-facing burpees.

Recommendations:
Deadlifts: Maintain proper form to protect your back. Break into manageable sets early to avoid burnout.
Bar-Facing Burpees: Maintain a steady pace and use efficient movement patterns.
Pacing: Start at a consistent, sustainable pace and aim to maintain it throughout the workout.

Workout 22.3

Workout:

For Time:

Time cap: 12 minutes

21 Pull-Ups
42 Double-Unders
21 Thrusters (43kg/95lbs for men, 29.5kg/65lbs for women)
18 Chest-to-Bar Pull-Ups
36 Double-Unders
18 Thrusters (52.5kg/115lbs for men, 35kg/75lbs for women)
15 Bar Muscle-Ups
30 Double-Unders
15 Thrusters (61kg/135lbs for men, 43kg/95lbs for women)

Description:
A combination of pull-ups, double-unders, and thrusters with increasing difficulty, testing your gymnastics skill, cardio capacity, and strength.

Recommendations:
Pull-Ups and Chest-to-Bar Pull-Ups: Break into manageable sets early to avoid grip fatigue. Use efficient kipping to save energy.
Bar Muscle-Ups: If proficient, aim for unbroken or small sets. Use efficient kipping to save energy.
Double-Unders: Aim for unbroken sets if proficient. Break into manageable sets if necessary to maintain rhythm.
Thrusters: Find a rhythm and pace that you can maintain. Break into manageable sets to avoid burning out.
Pacing: Move efficiently through each movement to save energy for the later parts of the workout.

2023 Open Workouts

Workout 23.1

Workout:

14-minute AMRAP

60 Calorie Row
50 Toes-to-Bar
40 Wall Balls (9kg/20lbs to 10 feet for men, 6kg/14lbs to 9 feet for women)
30 Clean and Jerks (61kg/135lbs for men, 43kg/95lbs for women)
20 Ring Muscle-Ups

Description:
A chipper workout testing your endurance, core strength, and gymnastic ability with a mix of rowing, toes-to-bar, wall balls, clean and jerks, and ring muscle-ups.

Recommendations:
Row: Maintain a consistent pace that allows you to recover while still keeping a strong output.
Toes-to-Bar: Break into manageable sets early to avoid grip fatigue. Use efficient kipping to save energy.
Wall Balls: Aim for unbroken sets if possible, or break into smaller sets with short rest.
Clean and Jerks: Use efficient technique and quick singles if necessary. Focus on maintaining good form.
Ring Muscle-Ups: If proficient, aim for unbroken or small sets. Use efficient kipping to save energy.

Pacing: Move efficiently through each movement to save energy for the later parts of the workout.

Workout 23.2A

Workout:

15-minute AMRAP

5 Burpee Pull-Ups
10 Shuttle Runs (1 rep = 25 feet out + 25 feet back)

Description:
A simple yet challenging combination of burpee pull-ups and shuttle runs, testing your cardio capacity and upper body endurance.

Recommendations:
Burpee Pull-Ups: Maintain a steady pace and use efficient movement patterns. Jump to a pull-up bar height that allows you to use momentum from the jump.
Shuttle Runs: Keep a steady pace, focusing on smooth turns at each end.
Pacing: Start at a consistent, sustainable pace and aim to maintain it throughout the workout.

Workout 23.2B

Workout:

Immediately following 23.2A, establish a 1-rep-max thruster

Time cap: 5 minutes

Description:

A strength test following a metabolic workout, testing your ability to lift under fatigue.

Recommendations:

Strategy: Plan your attempts. Start with a safe weight and make incremental increases. Allow enough rest between attempts to maximise your lifts.

Technique: Focus on maintaining good form and efficient movement patterns. Use the drive from the legs to assist the press.

Pacing: Use the 5 minutes wisely, planning for 2-3 attempts based on how fatigued you feel after 23.2A.

Workout 23.3

Workout:

Starting with a 6-minute time cap, complete as many reps as possible of:

If completed before the 6-minute time cap, add 3 minutes to the time cap and complete:

5 Wall Walks

50 Double-Unders

15 Snatches (43kg/95lbs for men, 29.5kg/65lbs for women)

5 Wall Walks

50 Double-Unders

12 Snatches (61kg/135lbs for men, 43kg/95lbs for women)

Description:

A workout with increasing difficulty, combining wall walks, double-unders, snatches, and strict handstand push-ups, testing your strength, skill, and endurance.

Recommendations:

Wall Walks: Maintain control and use efficient movement patterns. Rest briefly between reps if necessary.

Double-Unders: Aim for unbroken sets if proficient. Break into manageable sets if necessary to maintain rhythm.

Snatches: Use efficient technique and quick singles if necessary. Focus on maintaining good form as the weight increases.

Strict Handstand Push-Ups: Maintain a tight midline and use efficient movement patterns. Break into small sets early to avoid failure.

Pacing: Move efficiently through each movement to save energy for the later parts of the workout.

2024 Open Workouts

Workout 24.1

Workout:

For Time:

Time cap: 15 minutes

21 Dumbbell Snatches (22.5kg/50lbs for men, 15kg/35lbs for women) with one arm
21 Lateral Burpees over the Dumbbell
21 Dumbbell Snatches with the other arm
21 Lateral Burpees over the Dumbbell
15 Dumbbell Snatches with one arm

15 Lateral Burpees over the Dumbbell

15 Dumbbell Snatches with the other arm

15 Lateral Burpees over the Dumbbell

9 Dumbbell Snatches with one arm

9 Lateral Burpees over the Dumbbell

9 Dumbbell Snatches with the other arm

9 Lateral Burpees over the Dumbbell

Description:

This workout tests your strength, endurance, and ability to maintain a high pace with a mix of dumbbell snatches and lateral burpees over the dumbbell.

Recommendations:

Dumbbell Snatches: Use a smooth and efficient movement. Switch hands in the air to save time.

Lateral Burpees: Maintain a steady, controlled pace. Consider stepping down from the burpee to conserve energy.

Pacing: Start at a steady pace and aim to maintain it throughout the workout. Avoid going all out at the beginning to prevent early burnout.

Workout 24.2

Workout:

20-minute AMRAP

300-Meter Row

10 Deadlifts (84kg/185lbs for men, 57kg/125lbs for women)

50 Double-Unders

Description:

This workout combines rowing, deadlifts, and double-unders, testing your cardio capacity, strength, and coordination.

Recommendations:

Row: Maintain a consistent pace that allows you to recover while still keeping a strong output. Set the damper setting between 5 and 6, consistent with your usual practice.

Deadlifts: Maintain proper form to protect your back. Use a mixed grip and perform touch-and-go reps if possible.

Double-Unders: Aim for unbroken sets if proficient. Keep jumps controlled and use wrist movement to spin the rope.

Pacing: Start at a sustainable pace to avoid early fatigue. Manage your energy to maintain consistent round times.

Workout 24.3

Workout:

For Time:

5 rounds of:

10 thrusters (43kg/95lbs for men, 29.5kg/65lbs for women)
10 chest-to-bar pull-ups

Rest 1 minute, then:

5 rounds of:

7 thrusters (61kg/135lbs for men, 43kg/95lbs for women)
7 bar muscle-ups

Description:

This workout tests your endurance, strength, and gymnastic skills with a combination of thrusters, chest-to-bar pull-ups, and bar muscle-ups.

Recommendations:

Thrusters: Find a rhythm and pace that you can maintain. Break into manageable sets to avoid burning out.

Chest-to-Bar Pull-Ups: Use a kipping or butterfly technique to save your grip and shoulders. Break into smaller sets early to avoid failure.

Bar Muscle-Ups: If proficient, aim for unbroken or small sets. Use efficient kipping to save energy.

Pacing: Move efficiently through each movement to save energy for the later parts of the workout.

THE GIRLS

"The Girls" are a unique set of benchmark workouts introduced by CrossFit in 2003. These workouts are considered classic to the CrossFit community, often serving as key indicators of an athlete's progress over time. Each one is characterized by its intensity and wide range of movements.

Why are they named after women? According to CrossFit founder Greg Glassman, he named the workouts after women following the same convention used for naming hurricanes. He felt that because these workouts are so physically intense that they leave you feeling storm-tossed, it was appropriate to give them women's names.

Now, let's explore these classic CrossFit benchmarks:

Amanda For time 9-7-5:

- Muscle-ups

- Squat Snatches (135/96 lbs - 61/43 kg)

Angie For time:

- 100 pull-ups

- 100 push-ups

- 100 sit-ups

- 100 squats

Annie For time 50-40-30-20-10:

- Double-unders

- Sit-ups

Barbara Five rounds, each for time of:

- 20 pull-ups

- 30 push-ups

- 40 sit-ups

- 50 squats

- (Rest precisely three minutes between each round.)

Candy Five round for time:

- 20 pull-ups

- 30 push-ups

- 40 sit-ups

- 50 air squats

- 3 minute rest

Chelsea Every minute on the minute for 30 minutes:

- 5 pull-ups

- 10 push-ups

- 15 squats

Cindy AMRAP in 20 minutes:

- 5 pull-ups

- 10 push-ups

- 15 air squats

Diane For time:

- 21-15-9 reps of deadlifts (225/155 lbs - 102/70 kg)

- Handstand push-ups

Elizabeth For time:

- 21-15-9 reps of cleans (135/96 lbs - 61/43 kg)

- Ring dips

Eva Five round for time:

- 800m run

- 30 kettlebell swings (2 pood)

- 30 pull-ups

Fran For time:

- 21-15-9 reps of thrusters (95/65 lbs – 43/30 kg)

- Pull-ups

Grace For time:

- 30 clean and jerks (135/96 lbs - 61/43 kg)

Gwen Reps for load:

- Clean and jerks (unbroken)

- Rest as needed between sets

Helen Three rounds for time:

- 400-meter run

- 21 kettlebell swings (1.5/1 pood)

- 12 pull-ups

Isabel For time:

- 30 snatches (135/96 lbs - 61/43 kg)

Jackie For time:

- 1000 meter row

- 50 thrusters (45 lbs/20 kg)

- 30 pull-ups

Karen For time:

- 150 wall-ball shots (20/14 lbs - 9/6 kg)

Kelly Five round for time:

- 400m run

- 30 box jumps (24/20")

- 30 wall balls (20/14 lbs - 9/6 kg)

Linda (aka "3 bars of death") 10-9-8-7-6-5-4-3-2-1 reps for time of:

- Deadlift at 1.5 times body weight

- Bench press at body weight

- Clean at 3/4 body weight

Lynne Five rounds for max reps:

- Bench press (body weight)

- Pull-ups

Mary As many rounds as possible in 20 minutes:

- 5 handstand push-ups

- 10 one-legged squats, alternating

- 15 pull-ups

Nancy Five rounds for time:

- 400-meter run

- 15 overhead squats (95/65 lbs – 43/30 kg)

Nicole As many rounds as possible in 20 minutes:

- 400-meter run

- Max reps pull-ups

THE NEW GIRLS

As CrossFit has evolved and expanded, it introduced a second set of benchmark workouts, known as "The New Girls". Continuing in the tradition of the original Girls, these workouts test a broad range of physical capacities, from endurance and strength to agility and balance. They provide additional challenges for athletes and additional benchmarks to measure fitness progress.

Let's introduce The New Girls:

Andi For Time:

- 100 Hang Power Snatches (65/45 lbs - 29/20 kg)

- 100 Push Presses (65/45 lbs - 29/20 kg)

- 100 Sumo Deadlift High Pulls (65/45 lbs - 29/20 kg)

- 100 Front Squats (65/45 lbs - 29/20 kg)

Barbara Ann 5 Rounds for Time:

- 20 Handstand Push-Ups

- 30 Deadlifts (135/96 lbs - 61/43 kg)

- 40 Sit-Ups

- 50 Double-Unders

- 3-Minute Rest

Ellen 3 Rounds for Time:

- 20 Burpees

- 21 Dumbbell Snatches (50/35 lbs - 23/16 kg)

- 12 Dumbbell Thrusters (2x 50/35 lbs - 23/16 kg)

Grettel 10 Rounds for Time:

- 3 Clean-and-Jerks (135/96 lbs - 61/43 kg)

- 3 Burpees over the Bar

Lane 5 Rounds for Max Reps:

- ¾ Bodyweight Hang Power Snatches

- Handstand Push-Ups

- Rest as Needed Between Rounds

Lyla For Time:

- 10-1 Reps of Muscle-Ups

- Bodyweight Clean-and-Jerks

Ingrid 10 Rounds for Time:

- 3 Snatches (135/96 lbs - 61/43 kg)

- 3 Burpees over the Bar

Hero WODs

CrossFit is more than just a training methodology; it's a community that respects and honors the brave individuals who have paid the ultimate sacrifice in the line of duty. To commemorate these heroes, CrossFit has created a series of workouts known as "Hero WODs". Each workout is dedicated to a person who has lost their life serving their country or community.

Hero WODs are typically more challenging and longer than regular CrossFit workouts. They are designed not only to be physically demanding but also to test your mental strength and resilience, much like the heroes they're named after. As with all CrossFit workouts, it's important to scale appropriately and maintain proper form throughout.

Abbey Seven rounds for time:

- 50 Double-unders

- 20 Box jump-overs (24/20")

- 10 Handstand push-ups

Abbate For time:

- Run 1 mile

- 21 Clean and jerk (155/110 lbs - 70/50 kg)

- Run 800 meters

- 21 Clean and jerk (155/110 lbs - 70/50 kg)

- Run 1 Mile

Adam Brown Two rounds for time:

- 24 Deadlift (295/220 lbs - 134/100 kg)

- 24 Box jumps (24/20")

- 24 Wallball shots (20/14 lbs - 9/6 kg)

- 24 Bench press (195/143 lbs - 88/65 kg)

- 24 Box jumps (24/20")

- 24 Wallball shots (20/14 lbs - 9/6 kg)

- 24 Cleans (145/99 lbs - 66/45 kg)

Arnie With a single 2 pood kettlebell:

- 21 Turkish get-ups, Right arm

- 50 Swings

- 21 Overhead squats, Left arm

- 50 Swings

- 21 Overhead squats, Right arm

- 50 Swings

- 21 Turkish get-ups, Left arm

Badger Complete three rounds for time:

- 30 Squat cleans (95/65 lbs - 43/30 kg)

- 30 Pull-ups

- Run 800 meters

Blake Four rounds for time:

- 100 foot (~30 meters) Walking lunge with 45lb (20 kg) plate held overhead

- 30 Box jumps (24/20")

- 20 Wallball shots (20/14 lbs - 9/6 kg)

- 10 Handstand push-ups

Bradley 10 rounds for time:

- Sprint 100 meters

- 10 Pull-ups

- Sprint 100 meters

- 10 Burpees

- Rest 30 seconds

Brenton Five rounds for time:

- Bear crawl 100 feet (~30 meters)

- Standing broad-jump, 100 feet (~30 meters)
  (Do three Burpees after every five broad-jumps. If you've got
  a twenty-pound (~9 kg) vest or body armor, wear it.)

Bulger Ten rounds for time:

- Run 150 meters

- 7 Chest to bar pull-ups

- 7 Front squat (135/96 lbs - 61/43 kg)

- 7 Handstand push-ups

Carse 21-18-15-12-9-6-3 reps for time of:

- Squat clean (95/65 lbs - 43/30 kg)

- Double-under

- Deadlift (185/132 lbs - 84/60 kg)

- Box jump (24/20")

- Begin each round with a 50 meter Bear crawl

Coe Ten rounds for time:

- 10 Thrusters (95/65 lbs - 43/30 kg)

- 10 Ring push-ups

Collin Six rounds for time:

- Carry 50 pound (22 kg) sandbag 400 meters

- 12 Push press (115/81 lbs - 52/37 kg)

- 12 Box jumps (24/20")

- 12 Sumo deadlift high-pull (95/65 lbs - 43/30 kg)

Cory For time:

- Run 1 mile

- 100 Sit-ups

- 100 Back extensions

- 100 Squats

- Run 1 mile

Danny As many rounds in 20 minutes as you can of:

- 30 Box Jump (24/20")

- 20 Push Press (115/81 lbs - 52/37 kg)

- 30 Pull-ups

Del For time:

- 25 Burpees

- Run 400 meters with a 20 pound (9 kg) medicine ball

- 25 Weighted pull-ups with 20 pound dumbbell

- Run 400 meters with a 20 pound medicine ball

- 25 Handstand push-ups

- Run 400 meters with a 20 pound medicine ball

- 25 Chest-to-bar pull-ups

- Run 400 meters with a 20 pound medicine ball

- 25 Burpees

DG As many rounds as possible in 10 minutes of:

- 8 Toes-to-bar

- 35 pound (16 kg) Dumbbell thruster, 8 reps

- 35 pound (16 kg) Dumbbell walking lunge, 12 steps

Dork Six rounds for time of:

- 60 Double-unders

- 30 Kettlebell swings (2 pood)

- 15 Burpees

DT Five rounds for time:

- 12 Deadlifts (155/110 lbs - 70/50 kg)

- 9 Hang power cleans (155/110 lbs - 70/50 kg)

- 6 Push jerks (155/110 lbs - 70/50 kg)

Erin Five rounds for time:

- 15 Dumbbells split clean (40/27 lbs - 18/13 kg)

- 21 Pull-ups

Falkel As many rounds as possible in 25 minutes:

- 8 Handstand push-ups

- 8 Box Jump (30/24")

- 15 foot Rope climb, 1 ascent

Feeks For time:

- Run 1.5 miles

- 100 Push-ups

- 20 Back squat (155/110 lbs - 70/50 kg)

- Run 1.5 miles

Forrest Three rounds for time:

- 20 L-pull-ups

- 30 Toes to bar

- 40 Burpees

- Run 800 meters

Garrett Three rounds for time:

- 75 Squats

- 25 Ring handstand push-ups

- 25 L-pull-ups

Gator Eight rounds for time:

- 5 Front squat (185/132 lbs - 84/60 kg)

- 26 Ring push-ups

Gaza Five rounds for time:

- 35 Kettlebell swings (2 pood)

- 30 Push-ups

- 25 Pull-ups

- 20 Box jumps (30/24")

- 1-mile run

Glen For time:

- 30 Clean and jerks (135/96 lbs - 61/43 kg)

- Run 1 mile

- 10 Rope climbs

- Run 1 mile

- 100 Burpees

Griff For time:

- Run 800 meters

- Run 400 meters backwards

- Run 800 meters

- Run 400 meters backwards

Hammer Five rounds, each for time, of:

- 5 Power clean (135/96 lbs - 61/43 kg)

- 10 Front squat (135/96 lbs - 61/43 kg)

- 5 Jerk (135/96 lbs - 61/43 kg)

- 20 Pull-ups

- Rest 90 seconds

Hansen Five rounds for time:

- 30 Kettlebell swing (2 pood)

- 30 Burpees

- 30 Glute-ham sit-ups

Harper Complete as many rounds as possible in 23 minutes of:

- 9 Chest-to-bar pull-ups

- 15 Power clean (135/96 lbs - 61/43 kg)

- 21 Squats

- Run 400 meters with a 45 pound (20 kg) plate held overhead

Helton Three rounds for time:

- Run 800 meters

- 30 Dumbbell squat cleans (50/35 lbs - 23/16 kg)

- 30 Burpees

Hidalgo For time:

- Run 2 miles

- Rest 2 minutes

- 20 Squat cleans (50/35 lbs - 23/16 kg)

- 20 Box jump (24/20")

- 20 Walking lunge steps with 45lb plate held overhead

- 20 Box jump (24/20")

- 20 Squat cleans (135/96 lbs - 61/43 kg)

- Rest 2 minutes

- Run 2 miles

Holbrook Ten rounds, each for time:

- 5 Thruster (115/81 lbs - 52/37 kg)

- 10 Pull-ups

- 100 meter Sprint

- Rest 1 minute

Holleyman 30 rounds for time:

- 5 Wall ball shots (20/14 lbs - 9/6 kg)

- 3 Handstand push-ups

- 1 Power clean (225/155 lbs - 102/70 kg)

Hotshots 19 Six rounds for time:

- 30 Squats

- 19 Power cleans (135/96 lbs - 61/43 kg)

- 7 Strict Pull-ups

- Run 400 meters

Ivan the Terrible Three rounds for time:

- Run 400 meters

- 50 Pull-ups

- Run 400 meters

- 50 Push-ups

- Run 400 meters

- 50 Sit-ups

- Run 400 meters

- 50 Squats

Jack As many rounds as possible in 20 minutes:

- 10 Push press (115/81 lbs - 52/37 kg)

- 10 Kettlebell swings (1.5 pood)

- 10 Box jumps (24/20")

Jag 28 For time:

- Run 800 meters

- 28 Kettlebell swings (2 pood)

- 28 Strict Pull-ups

- 28 Kettlebell clean and jerk (2 pood)

- 28 Strict Pull-ups

- Run 800 meters

Jared Four rounds for time:

- Run 800 meters

- 40 Pull-ups

- 70 Push-ups

Jason For time:

- 100 Squats

- 5 Muscle-ups

- 75 Squats

- 10 Muscle-ups

- 50 Squats

- 15 Muscle-ups

- 25 Squats

- 20 Muscle-ups

JBo Complete as many rounds as possible in 28 minutes of:

- 9 Overhead squats (115/81 lbs - 52/37 kg)

- 1 Legless rope climb (15 ft / ~4.5 meters)

- 12 Bench presses (115/81 lbs - 52/37 kg)

Jenny As many rounds as possible in 20 minutes of:

- 20 Overhead squats (45 lbs / 20 kg)

- 20 Back squats (45 lbs / 20 kg)

- 400-meter run

Jerry For time:

- Run 1 mile

- Row 2K

- Run 1 mile

J.J. For time:

- 1 Squat clean (185/132 lbs - 84/60 kg)

- 10 Parallette handstand push-ups

- 2 Squat clean (185/132 lbs - 84/60 kg)

- 9 Parallette handstand push-ups

- 3 Squat clean(185/132 lbs - 84/60 kg)

- 8 Parallette handstand push-ups
  ... Continue this pattern until the final round of 10 squat cleans and 1 handstand push-up.

Josh For time:

- 21 Overhead squats (95/65 lbs - 43/30 kg)

- 42 Pull-ups

- 15 Overhead squats (95/65 lbs - 43/30 kg)

- 30 Pull-ups

- 9 Overhead squats (95/65 lbs - 43/30 kg)

- 18 Pull-ups

Joshie Three rounds for time of:

- 40-pound (18 kg) Dumbbell snatch, 21 reps, right arm

- 21 L pull-ups

- 40-pound (18 kg) Dumbbell snatch, 21 reps, left arm

- 21 L pull-ups

JT For time:

- 21-15-9 reps of:

- Handstand push-ups

- Ring dips

- Push-ups

Justin For time:

- 30-20-10 reps of:

- Bodyweight back squats

- Bodyweight bench presses

- Strict pull-ups

Kalsu For time:

- 100 Thrusters (135/96 lbs - 61/43 kg)

- Begin each minute with 5 burpees, then complete as many thrusters as possible during the remainder of the minute. Repeat until 100 total thrusters are completed.

Kenny For time:

- 50 Double unders

- 10 Thrusters (135/96 lbs - 61/43 kg)

- 15 Thrusters (95/65 lbs - 43/30 kg)

- 20 Thrusters (65/45 lbs - 29/20 kg)

- 50 Double unders

Kevin Three rounds for time:

- 32 Deadlifts (185/132 lbs - 84/60 kg)

- 32 Hanging hip touches

- 800-meter Run

King Kong Three rounds for time:

- 1 Deadlift (455 lbs / 206 kg)

- 2 Muscle-ups

- 3 Squat Cleans (250 lbs / 113 kg)

- 4 Handstand Push-ups

Klepto Four rounds for time:

- 27 Box jumps (24/20")

- 20 Burpees

- 11 Squat cleans (145/99 lbs - 66/45 kg)

Kutschbach Seven rounds for time:

- 11 Back squats (185/132 lbs - 84/60 kg)

- 10 Jerks (135/96 lbs - 61/43 kg)

Ledesma As many rounds as possible in 20 minutes:

- 5 Parallette handstand push-ups (10 inch / ~25 cm deficit)

- 10 Toes through rings

- 15 Medicine ball cleans (20/14 lbs - 9/6 kg)

Loredo Six rounds for time:

- 24 Squats

- 24 Push-ups

- 24 Walking lunge steps

- Run 400 meters

Luce Three rounds for time:

- 1K Run

- 10 Muscle-ups

- 100 Squats

Luke For time:

- 400-meter Run

- 15 Clean and jerks (155/110 lbs - 70/50 kg)

- 400-meter Run

- 30 Toes-to-bars

- 400-meter Run

- 45 Wall-ball shots (20/14 lbs - 9/6 kg)

- 400-meter Run

- 45 Kettlebell swings (1.5 pood)

- 400-meter Run

- 30 Ring dips

- 400-meter Run

- 15 Weighted lunges (155/110 lbs - 70/50 kg)

- 400-meter Run

Manion Seven rounds for time:

- Run 400 meters

- 29 Back squats

Marco Three rounds for time:

- 21 Pull-ups

- 15 Handstand push-ups

- 9 Thrusters (135/96 lbs - 61/43 kg)

McCluskey Three rounds for time:

- 9 Muscle-ups

- 15 Burpee pull-ups

- 21 Pull-ups

- Run 800 meters

McGhee As many rounds as possible in 30 minutes:

- 275 pound (125 kg) Deadlift, 5 reps

- 13 Push-ups

- 9 Box jumps (24/20")

McLaren For time:

- 1000 meter Row

- 200 Double-unders

- 50 Alternating pistols

- 30 Hang power cleans (185/132 lbs - 84/60 kg)

Michael Three rounds for time:

- Run 800 meters

- 50 Back Extensions

- 50 Sit-ups

Moon Seven rounds for time:

- 40 pound (18 kg) Dumbbell hang split snatch, 10 reps Right arm

- 15 ft Rope Climb, 1 ascent

- 40 pound (18 kg) Dumbbell hang split snatch, 10 reps Left arm

- 15 ft Rope Climb, 1 ascent

Moore As many rounds as possible in 20 minutes:

- 15 ft Rope Climb, 1 ascent

- Run 400 meters

- Max rep Handstand push-ups

Morrison 50-40-30-20-10 reps for time:

- Wall ball shots (20/14 lbs - 9/6 kg)

- Box jumps (24/20")

- Kettlebell swings (1.5 pood)

Mr. Joshua Five rounds for time:

- Run 400 meters

- 30 Glute-ham sit-ups

- 15 Deadlifts (250 lbs / 113 kg)

Murph For time:

- Run 1 mile

- 100 Pull-ups

- 200 Push-ups

- 300 Squats

- Run 1 mile

Nate As many rounds as possible in 20 minutes:

- 2 Muscle-ups

- 4 Handstand push-ups

- 8 Kettlebell swings (2 pood)

Nautical Nancy Five rounds for time:

- 500 Meter row

- 15 Overhead squats (95/65 lbs - 43/30 kg)

Ned Seven rounds for time:

- 11 Bodyweight back squats

- 1,000-meter row

Nutts For time:

- 10 Handstand push-ups

- 15 Deadlifts (250 lbs / ~113 kg)

- 25 Box jumps (30/24")

- 50 Pull-ups

- 100 Wall-ball shots (20/14 lbs - 9/6 kg)

- 200 Double-unders

- Run 400 meters with a 45 lbs (~20 kg) plate

Ozzy As many rounds as possible in 20 minutes:

- 11 Plate burpees (45 lbs / ~20 kg)

- 7 Strict pull-ups

- 400 Meter run

Paul Five rounds for time:

- 50 Double-unders

- 35 Knees-to-elbows

- 185 pound (84 kg) Overhead walk, 20 yards

Pheezy Three rounds for time:

- Five front squats (165 lbs / 75 kg)

- 18 Pull-ups

- 12 Burpees

Rahoi As many rounds as possible in 12 minutes:

- 12 Box jumps (24/20")

- 6 Thrusters (95/65 lbs - 43/30 kg)

- 6 Bar-facing burpees

Rankel As many rounds as possible in 20 minutes:

- 6 Deadlifts (225/155 lbs - 102/70 kg)

- 7 Burpee pull-ups

- 10 Kettlebell swings (2 pood)

- 200 meter Run

Randy For time:

- 75 Power snatches (75 lbs / ~34 kg)

Ricky As many rounds as possible in 20 minutes:

- 10 Pull-ups

- 75 pound (34 kg) Dumbbell Deadlift, 5 reps

- 135 pound (61 kg) Push-press, 8 reps

Roney Four rounds for time:

- 200 meter Run

- 11 Thruster (135/96 lbs - 61/43 kg)

- 200 meter Run

- 11 Push press (135/96 lbs - 61/43 kg)

- 200 meter Run

- 11 Bench press (135/96 lbs - 61/43 kg)

Roy Five rounds for time:

- 15 Deadlifts (225/155 lbs - 102/70 kg)

- 20 Box jumps (24/20")

- 25 Pull-ups

Ryan Five rounds for time:

- 7 Muscle-ups

- 21 Burpees

Santora Three rounds for reps:

- 155 pound (70 kg) Squat cleans, 1 minute

- 20' Shuttle sprints (20' forward + 20' backwards = 1 rep), 1 minute

- 245 pound (111 kg) Deadlifts, 1 minute

- Burpees, 1 minute

- 155 pound (70 kg) Jerks, 1 minute

- Rest 1 minute

Schmalls For time:

- Run 800 meters

- Then two rounds of:

  - 50 Burpees

  - 40 Pull-ups

  - 30 One-legged squats

  - 20 Kettlebell swings (1.5 pood)

  - 10 Handstand push-ups

- Then,

- Run 800 meters

Severin For time:

- 50 Strict Pull-ups

- 100 Push-ups, release hands from floor at the bottom

- Run 5K

Ship Nine rounds for time:

- 7 Squat cleans (185/132 lbs - 84/60 kg)

- 8 Burpee box jumps (36")

Sisson As many rounds as possible in 20 minutes:

- 15-ft Rope Climb, 1 ascent

- 5 Burpees

- 200 meter Run

Small Three rounds for time:

- Row 1000 meters

- 50 Burpees

- 50 Box jumps (24/20")

- Run 800 meters

Spehar For time:

- 100 Thrusters (135/96 lbs - 61/43 kg)

- 100 Chest-to-bar pull-ups

- Run 6 miles

Stephen 30-25-20-15-10-5 reps for time:

- GHD sit-ups

- Back extensions

- Knees to elbows

- 95 pound (43 kg) Stiff legged deadlift

Stevens Five rounds for time:

- Run 200 meters

- 50 pound (23 kg) Dumbbell snatch, 15 reps

- Run 200 meters

- 50 pound (23 kg) Dumbbell snatch, 15 reps

- Rest 1 minute

Stratton Ten rounds for time:

- 12 Burpees

- 12 Pull-ups

Taylor Four rounds for time:

- Run 400 meters

- 5 Burpee muscle-ups

The Seven Seven rounds for time:

- 7 Handstand push-ups

- 7 Thrusters (135/96 lbs - 61/43 kg)

- 7 Knees to elbows

- 7 Deadlifts (245 lbs / 111 kg)

- 7 Burpees

- 7 Kettlebell swings (2 pood)

- 7 Pull-ups

Thompson Ten rounds for time:

- 15 ft Rope Climb, 1 ascent

- 29 Back squats (95/65 lbs - 43/30 kg)

- 10 Steps barbell farmers carry (135/96 lbs - 61/43 kg)

- 15 ft Rope Climb, 1 ascent

- 10 Steps barbell farmers carry (135/96 lbs - 61/43 kg)

- 29 Back squats (95/65 lbs - 43/30 kg)

Tillman Seven rounds for time:

- 7 Deadlifts (315 lbs / ~143 kg)

- 1 Full gasser

- 15 Pull-ups

- 45 pound (20 kg) plate carry, 100 meters

Tumilson Eight rounds for time:

- Run 200 meters

- 11 Dumbbell burpee deadlifts (60 lbs / 27 kg)

Viola As many rounds as possible in 20 minutes:

- Run 400 meters

- 11 Power snatches (95/65 lbs - 43/30 kg)

- 17 Pull-ups

- 13 Power cleans (135/96 lbs - 61/43 kg)

Wes For time:

- Run 800 meters with a 25-pound (11 kg) plate

- Then, 14 rounds of:

    ○ 5 Strict pull-ups

    ○ 4 Burpee box jumps (24/20″)

    ○ 3 Cleans (185/132 lbs - 84/60 kg)

- Then, run 800 meters with a 25-pound (11 kg) plate

White Five rounds for time:

- 3 Rope climbs

- 10 Toes-to-bars

- 21 Walking lunge steps with 45lb (20 kg) plate overhead

- Run 400 meters

Wilmot Six rounds for time:

- 50 Squats

- 25 Ring dips

Wood Five rounds for time:

- Run 400 meters

- 10 Burpee box jumps (24/20")

- 95 pound (43 kg) Sumo-deadlift high-pull, 10 reps

- 95 pound (43 kg) Thruster, 10 reps

- Rest 1 minute

Wittman Seven rounds for time:

- 15 Kettlebell swings (1.5 pood)

- 15 Power cleans (95/65 lbs - 43/30 kg)

- 15 Box jumps (24/20")

Zembiec Five rounds for time:

- 11 Back squats (185/132 lbs - 84/60 kg)

- 7 Strict burpee pull-ups

- 400 meter Run

Zimmermann For time:

- 11 Chest-to-bar pull-ups

- 2 Deadlifts (315 lbs / 143 kg)

- 10 Chest-to-bar pull-ups

- 4 Deadlifts (315 lbs / 143 kg)

- 9 Chest-to-bar pull-ups

- 6 Deadlifts (315 lbs / 143 kg)

- 8 Chest-to-bar pull-ups

- 8 Deadlifts (315 lbs / 143 kg)

- 7 Chest-to-bar

BODYWEIGHT ONLY
WORKOUTS

In the realm of fitness, there's a popular saying: "Your body is your first gym." And for a good reason. Bodyweight exercises offer an incredibly versatile and accessible method of training that you can carry out virtually anywhere, anytime, and without any equipment.

While bodyweight exercises may seem simple, they provide a formidable challenge for both beginners and seasoned athletes. Relying solely on the weight of your body, these exercises can improve strength, flexibility, balance, and endurance, ensuring a comprehensive full-body workout.

Bodyweight workouts also form a crucial part of CrossFit training. From classic movements like push-ups, pull-ups, and squats to more advanced exercises like handstand push-ups and muscle-ups, these workouts will push your limits and help you discover the true potential of your body.

Whether you're training at home, in a hotel, at a park, or even in a full-scale gym, these bodyweight workouts provide an efficient way to get fit and stay in shape. The only equipment you need is your body, a good dose of determination, and perhaps a pull-up bar for certain workouts. So, let's dive in and explore the power of bodyweight training.

Invisible Ibex For Time:

- 100 Alternating Lunges

- 80 Sit-ups

- 60 Push-ups

- 40 Air Squats

- 20 Burpees

Rapid Rabbit 5 Rounds for Time:

- 20 Burpees

- 40 Air Squats

- 60 Jumping Jacks

Skipping Skunk For Time:

- 100-90-80-70-60-50-40-30-20-10 reps of Double-Unders and Sit-ups

Tumbling Tiger 3 Rounds for Time:

- 10 Handstand Push-ups

- 20 Jumping Lunges

- 30 Sit-ups

- 40 Double-Unders

Aerobic Antelope For Time:

- 100 Burpees

- 200 Double-Unders

- 300 Air Squats

Bear Crawl Burn 5 Rounds for Time:

- 100-meter Bear Crawl

- 30 Push-ups

Climbing Cobra For Time:

- 10-9-8-7-6-5-4-3-2-1 Reps of Handstand Push-ups

- 1-2-3-4-5-6-7-8-9-10 Reps of Broad Jumps

Dashing Deer For Time:

- 200 Air Squats

- 100 Sit-ups

- 50 Handstand Push-ups

Chasing Cheetah AMRAP in 20 minutes:

- 10 Push-ups

- 15 Hollow Rocks

- 20 Alternating Lunges

Elevated Eagle AMRAP in 20 minutes:

- 5 Pull-ups

- 10 Push-ups

- 15 Air Squats

Fleet-footed Fox 3 Rounds for Time:

- 800 meter Run

- 50 Push-ups

Flying Falcon For Time:

- 10 Rounds of 10 Push-ups, 10 Squats, 10 Sit-ups

Galloping Gazelle For Time:

- 150 Burpees

Descending Dragon For Time:

- Start with 10 Burpees, then each round reduce by 1

- Start with 1 Push-up, then each round increase by 1

Grassy Gazelle 4 Rounds for Time:

- Run 400 meters

- 50 Air Squats

Accelerated Apex For Time:

- 100 Double-Unders

- 75 Air Squats

- 50 Push-ups

- 25 Burpees

- 100 Double-Unders

Ascending Peaks For Time:

- 100 Double-Unders

- 90 Sit-ups

- 80 Alternating Lunges

- 70 Burpees

- 60 Push-ups

- 50 Air Squats

- 40 Hollow Rocks

- 30 Handstand Push-ups

- 20 Broad Jumps

- 10 Muscle-ups

Hopping Hare For Time:

- 100 Jumping Jacks

- 75 Air Squats

- 50 Push-ups

- 25 Burpees

Hurdling Hawk AMRAP in 20 minutes:

- 5 Pull-ups

- 10 Push-ups

- 15 Air Squats

Inverted Iguana AMRAP in 15 minutes:

- 5 Handstand Push-ups

- 10 Pistols (alternating legs)

- 15 V-ups

Jumping Jaguar 3 Rounds for Time:

- 200 Double-Unders

- 50 Sit-ups

- 25 Push-ups

Kangaroo 4 Rounds for Time:

- 15 Burpees

- 30 Air Squats

- 60 Double-Unders (or 120 Single-Unders)

Leaping Lizard For Time:

- 100 Lunges

- 80 Sit-ups

- 60 Push-ups

- 40 Jump Squats

- 20 Burpees

Mountain Goat 3 Rounds for Time:

- Run 800 meters

- 50 Mountain Climbers

Nimble Ninja AMRAP in 20 minutes:

- 5 Handstand Push-ups

- 10 Tuck Jumps

- 15 Sit-ups

- 20 Air Squats

Ostrich 5 Rounds for Time:

- 400 meter Run

- 50 Air Squats

Whirling Wolf AMRAP in 15 minutes:

- 10 Handstand Push-ups

- 20 Hollow Rocks

- 30 Air Squats

Xenial Xerus For Time:

- 50 Burpees

- 100 Push-ups

- 150 Air Squats

Penguin Waddle For Time:

- 100m Bear Crawl

- 100 Air Squats

- 100 Sit-ups

- 100m Bear Crawl

Bounding Bobcat 4 Rounds for Time:

- 400 meter Run

- 50 Air Squats

Quicksilver Quetzal AMRAP in 15 minutes:

- 5 Burpees

- 10 Push-ups

- 15 Air Squats

- 20 Sit-ups

Unseen Unicorn AMRAP in 20 minutes:

- 5 Pull-ups

- 10 Push-ups

- 15 Air Squats

Vaulting Viper For Time:

- 100 Air Squats

- 80 Sit-ups

- 60 Alternating Lunges

- 40 Push-ups

- 20 Burpees

Yielding Yak 5 Rounds for Time:

- Run 400 meters

- 30 Air Squats

- 20 Push-ups

- 10 Burpees

Zigzag Zebra For Time:

- 10-20-30-40-50-40-30-20-10 reps of Air Squats and Sit-ups

DUMBBELL WORKOUTS

Welcome to the realm of dumbbells! Dumbbells are a fantastic tool for strength and conditioning, offering a unique range of motion and versatility that can't be found in barbells alone. This section of our guide dives into the world of dumbbell-only workouts, where every WOD (Workout of the Day) will harness the power of this piece of equipment.

Dumbbell workouts are incredibly beneficial for building strength and muscle symmetry. They require each side of your body to work independently, which can help correct any imbalances and promote motor learning. Dumbbells are also very accessible, making them a great option for home workouts when you can't make it to the gym.

Whether you're a seasoned CrossFit athlete looking to challenge yourself in new ways, or a beginner seeking to incorporate weight training into your routine, dumbbell-only workouts can provide the variety and intensity you need.

In this chapter, we'll explore a range of workouts that use only dumbbells. From classic movements like dumbbell snatches, thrusters, and lunges, to more complex sequences, these WODs will challenge your strength, balance, and coordination.

Get ready to grab a pair of dumbbells and dive into these workouts that are sure to test your mettle and build your strength in ways you never thought possible. Let's get lifting!

Eagle's Eye 4 Rounds for Time:

- 12 Dumbbell Clean and Jerks (2x 50/35 lbs - 23/16 kg)

- 24 Double Unders

Falcon's Flight AMRAP in 20 minutes:

- 5 Dumbbell Man Makers (2x 50/35 lbs - 23/16 kg)

- 10 Box Jumps (24/20")

Galactic Grind 5 Rounds for Time:

- 15 Dumbbell Front Squats (2x 50/35 lbs - 23/16 kg)

- 30 Double Unders

Hawkeye's Hunt 3 Rounds for Time:

- 10 Dumbbell Thrusters (2x 50/35 lbs - 23/16 kg)

- 200 meter Run

Icarus' Impact For Time:

- 21-15-9 Reps of:

- Dumbbell Snatches (50/35 lbs - 23/16 kg)

- Pull-ups

Jaguar's Jaunt AMRAP in 15 minutes:

- 15 Dumbbell Deadlifts (2x 50/35 lbs - 23/16 kg)

- 15 Push-ups

Kestrel's Kettle 5 Rounds for Time:

- 10 Dumbbell Overhead Lunges (2x 50/35 lbs - 23/16 kg)

- 10 Burpees

Lion's Leap For Time:

- 100 Dumbbell Goblet Squats (50/35 lbs - 23/16 kg)
  *Every minute on the minute, perform 5 burpees.

Mammoth's March 4 Rounds for Time:

- 12 Dumbbell Hang Clean and Jerks (2x 50/35 lbs - 23/16 kg)

- 24 Sit-ups

Night Owl AMRAP in 12 minutes:

- 12 Dumbbell Push Presses (2x 50/35 lbs - 23/16 kg)

- 12 Box Jumps (24/20")

Operation Overhead 5 Rounds for Time:

- 12 Dumbbell Push Presses (2x 50/35 lbs - 23/16 kg)

- 16 Alternating Dumbbell Lunges (2x 50/35 lbs - 23/16 kg)

- 20 Double Unders

Pinnacle Peaks For Time:

- 100 Dumbbell Thrusters (2x 50/35 lbs - 23/16 kg)
  *Every minute on the minute, perform 5 burpees.

Quicksilver Quest AMRAP in 20 minutes:

- 5 Dumbbell Man Makers (2x 50/35 lbs - 23/16 kg)

- 10 Toes-to-bars

- 15 Box Jumps (24/20 in)

Rapid Rivers 3 Rounds for Time:

- 15 Dumbbell Deadlifts (2x 50/35 lbs - 23/16 kg)

- 15 Dumbbell Hang Power Cleans (2x 50/35 lbs - 23/16 kg)

- 15 Dumbbell Push Presses (2x 50/35 lbs - 23/16 kg)

- 15 Devil Press (2x 50/35 lbs - 23/16 kg)

- 200 meter Run

Stellar Storm For Time:

- 21-15-9 Reps of:

- Dumbbell Snatches (50/35 lbs - 23/16 kg)

- Pull-ups

- Double Unders

Titan's Torment AMRAP in 15 minutes:

- 10 Dumbbell Thrusters (2x 50/35 lbs - 23/16 kg)

- 15 Dumbbell Swings (50/35 lbs - 23/16 kg)

- 20 Sit-ups

Unseen Universe 5 Rounds for Time:

- 10 Dumbbell Overhead Lunges (2x 50/35 lbs - 23/16 kg)

- 15 Dumbbell Deadlifts (2x 50/35 lbs - 23/16 kg)

- 20 Double Unders

Vortex Voyage For Time:

- 50 Dumbbell Front Squats (2x 50/35 lbs - 23/16 kg)

- 40 Dumbbell Push Presses (2x 50/35 lbs - 23/16 kg)

- 30 Dumbbell Snatches (2x 50/35 lbs - 23/16 kg)

- 20 Dumbbell Goblet Squats (50/35 lbs - 23/16 kg)

- 10 Dumbbell Man Makers (2x 50/35 lbs - 23/16 kg)

Whirlwind's Whim 4 Rounds for Time:

- 12 Dumbbell Hang Clean and Jerks (2x 50/35 lbs - 23/16 kg)

- 24 Double Unders

- 36 Sit-ups

Xenon X-factor AMRAP in 12 minutes:

- 12 Dumbbell Push Presses (2x 50/35 lbs - 23/16 kg)

- 12 Dumbbell Deadlifts (2x 50/35 lbs - 23/16 kg)

- 12 Box Jumps (24/20")

Hollow Dreams 3 Rounds for Time:

- 15 Dumbbell Hang Cleans (2x 50/35 lbs - 23/16 kg)

- 20 Push-ups

- 25 Air Squats

Spartan Sprint For Time:

- 50-40-30-20-10

- Dumbbell Deadlifts (2x 50/35 lbs - 23/16 kg)

- Double Unders

Jupiter's Grasp 5 Rounds for Time:

- 10 Dumbbell Thrusters (2x 50/35 lbs - 23/16 kg)

- 15 Box Jumps (24/20")

Olympus Odyssey AMRAP in 18 minutes:

- 12 Dumbbell Snatches (2x 50/35 lbs - 23/16 kg)

- 16 Toes-to-bars

- 20 Double Unders

Viper Venom 4 Rounds for Time:

- 15 Dumbbell Swings (50/35 lbs - 23/16 kg)

- 15 Burpees

- 200 meter Run

Time Traveler For Time:

- 21-15-9

- Dumbbell Front Squats (2x 50/35 lbs - 23/16 kg)

- Pull-ups

Dumbbell DT 5 Rounds for Time:

- 12 Cleans (2x 50/35 lbs - 23/16 kg)

- 9 Front Squats (2x 50/35 lbs - 23/16 kg)

- 6 Should to Overhead (2x 50/35 lbs - 23/16 kg)

Cosmic Crusader For Time:

- 50 Dumbbell Push Presses (2x 50/35 lbs - 23/16 kg)

- 40 Dumbbell Lunges (2x 50/35 lbs - 23/16 kg)

- 30 Dumbbell Deadlifts (2x 50/35 lbs - 23/16 kg)

- 20 Dumbbell Snatches (2x 50/35 lbs - 23/16 kg)

- 10 Dumbbell Goblet Squats (50/35 lbs - 23/16 kg)

Polaris Path 5 Rounds for Time:

- 12 Dumbbell Hang Clean and Jerks (2x 50/35 lbs - 23/16 kg)

- 24 Double Unders

- 36 Sit-ups

Asteroid's Anguish AMRAP in 12 minutes:

- 15 Dumbbell Push Presses (2x 50/35 lbs - 23/16 kg)

- 15 Box Jumps (24/20 in)

Neptune's Nemesis 4 Rounds for Time:

- 10 Dumbbell Thrusters (2x 50/35 lbs - 23/16 kg)

- 20 Dumbbell Deadlifts (2x 50/35 lbs - 23/16 kg)

- 30 Double Unders

Comet's Curse AMRAP in 16 minutes:

- 5 Dumbbell Man Makers (2x 50/35 lbs - 23/16 kg)

- 10 Toes-to-bars

- 15 Box Jumps (24/20")

Solar Surge 5 Rounds for Time:

- 12 Dumbbell Push Presses (2x 50/35 lbs - 23/16 kg)

- 16 Alternating Dumbbell Lunges (2x 50/35 lbs - 23/16 kg)

- 20 Double Unders

Galactic Grind For Time:

- 100 Dumbbell Thrusters (2x 50/35 lbs - 23/16 kg)
  *Every minute on the minute, perform 5 burpees

Orion's Orbit 4 Rounds for Time:

- 10 Dumbbell Devil's Press (2x 50/35 lbs - 23/16 kg)

- 20 Sit-ups

- 30 Double Unders

Meteor Mayhem For Time:

- 50-40-30-20-10

- Dumbbell Snatches (50/35 lbs - 23/16 kg)

- Wall Balls (20/14 lbs - 9/6 kg)

Pegasus Pursuit AMRAP in 15 minutes:

- 12 Dumbbell Goblet Squats (50/35 lbs - 23/16 kg)

- 16 Dumbbell Lunges (2x 50/35 lbs - 23/16 kg)

- 20 Double Unders

Saturn's Stride 5 Rounds for Time:

- 15 Dumbbell Deadlifts (2x 50/35 lbs - 23/16 kg)

- 15 Burpees to Bar

- 15 Wall Walks

Ursa Unleashed For Time:

- 21-15-9

- Dumbbell Thrusters (2x 50/35 lbs - 23/16 kg)

- Pull-ups

Venus Vortex AMRAP in 12 minutes:

- 10 Dumbbell Hang Clean and Jerks (2x 50/35 lbs - 23/16 kg)

- 20 Air Squats

Andromeda Assault 3 Rounds for Time:

- 15 Dumbbell Swings (50/35 lbs - 23/16 kg)

- 30 Sit-ups (RX+ GHD Sit-ups or weighted)

Celestial Charge For Time:

- 100 Dumbbell Snatches (50/35 lbs - 23/16 kg)
  *Every minute on the minute, perform 5 burpees.

Nebula Nexus AMRAP in 20 minutes:

- 5 Dumbbell Man Makers (2x 50/35 lbs - 23/16 kg)

- 10 Toes-to-bars

- 15 Box Jumps (24/20")

Solar Storm 5 Rounds for Time:

- 12 Dumbbell Push Presses (2x 50/35 lbs - 23/16 kg)

- 16 Alternating Dumbbell Lunges (2x 50/35 lbs - 23/16 kg)

- 20 Double Unders

Dumbbell Khaos AMRAP in 15 minutes:

- 15 Dumbbell Push Presses (2x 50/35 lbs - 23/16 kg)

- 10 Dumbbell Overhead Squats Left (50/35 lbs - 23/16 kg)

- 10 Dumbbell Overhead Squats Right (50/35 lbs - 23/16 kg)

- 30 Double Unders

Lever Lift 4 Rounds for Time:

- 12 Dumbbell Deadlifts (2x 50/35 lbs - 23/16 kg)

- 12 Dumbbell Hang Cleans (2x 50/35 lbs - 23/16 kg)

- 12 Dumbbell Push Presses (2x 50/35 lbs - 23/16 kg)

Mountaineer's Mile 5 Rounds for Time:

- 10 Dumbbell Snatches (50/35 lbs - 23/16 kg)

- 200 meter Run

Nimble Navigation 3 Rounds for Time:

- 400 meter Run

- 21 Dumbbell Swings (50/35 lbs - 23/16 kg)

Olympian Odyssey For Time:

- 30 Dumbbell Hang Power Cleans (2x 50/35 lbs - 23/16 kg)

- 30 Dumbbell Front Squats (2x 50/35 lbs - 23/16 kg)

- 30 Dumbbell Push Jerks (2x 50/35 lbs - 23/16 kg)

Peak Performance AMRAP in 20 minutes:

- 5 Devil Press (2x 50/35 lbs - 23/16 kg)

- 10 Dumbbell Overhead Lunges (2x 50/35 lbs - 23/16 kg)

- 15 Dumbbell Front Squats (2x 50/35 lbs - 23/16 kg)

Quasar Quest 3 Rounds for Time:

- 20 Dumbbell Thrusters (2x 50/35 lbs - 23/16 kg)

- 60 Double Unders

Rapid Resistance For Time:

- 21-15-9 Reps of:

- Dumbbell Deadlifts (2x 50/35 lbs - 23/16 kg)

- Dumbbell Power Cleans (2x 50/35 lbs - 23/16 kg)

- Dumbbell Push Presses (2x 50/35 lbs - 23/16 kg)

Stellar Strength For Time:

- 50 Dumbbell Hang Clean and Jerks (2x 50/35 lbs - 23/16

kg)

- Every minute, perform 5 Burpees

Titanium Tenacity 4 Rounds for Time:

- 12 Dumbbell Deadlifts (2x 50/35 lbs - 23/16 kg)

- 12 Dumbbell Overhead Lunges (2(2x 50/35 lbs - 23/16 kg)

- 12 Dumbbell Thrusters (2x 50/35 lbs - 23/16 kg)

KETTLEBELL WORKOUTS

The kettlebell, a weight resembling a cannonball with a handle, is a versatile and effective tool that has a place in any well-rounded fitness program. Originating in Russia, kettlebells have long been a staple in functional fitness and strength training, and for a good reason. Kettlebells are not only great for building strength and power, but they can also improve balance, agility, and coordination. They also allow for a wide range of movements that can be combined into complex workouts.

In CrossFit and Cross Training, kettlebell workouts are a staple. They can provide a full-body workout that challenges both your strength and cardiovascular system. Kettlebells are particularly effective at developing core and posterior chain strength, key areas for overall athletic performance.

This chapter will cover a wide range of workouts that only require a kettlebell. From simple yet challenging exercises like kettlebell swings, snatches, and cleans, to more complex flows that incorporate a sequence of movements, these workouts will push your fitness to new levels. Whether you're looking to improve your strength, conditioning, or both, there's a kettlebell workout in here for you.

Remember, as with any other workout, form and technique are crucial for kettlebell exercises. Always prioritize quality of movement over speed or volume. Now, let's swing into action!

Avalanche For Time:

- 100 Kettlebell Swings (53/35 lbs - 24/16 kg)

- Every minute on the minute, perform 5 Goblet Squats (53/35 lbs - 24/16 kg)

Bell Tower 5 Rounds for Time:

- 20 Kettlebell Snatches (10 each arm) (35/22 lbs - 16/10 kg)

- 20 Kettlebell Lunges (10 each leg) (35/22 lbs - 16/10 kg)

Iron Grip 21-15-9 reps for Time:

- Kettlebell Swings (53/35 lbs - 24/16 kg)

- Kettlebell Thrusters (2x 53/35 lbs - 24/16 kg)

Rapid Rapids 3 Rounds for Time:

- 400 meter Run

- 30 Kettlebell Clean and Press (15 each arm) (53/35 lbs - 24/16 kg)

Summit Climb AMRAP in 20 minutes:

- 10 Kettlebell Snatches (53/35 lbs - 24/16 kg)

- 15 Kettlebell Goblet Squats (53/35 lbs - 24/16 kg)

- 20 Kettlebell Swings (53/35 lbs - 24/16 kg)

Titan's Challenge 4 Rounds for Time:

- 20 Kettlebell Swings (70/53 lbs - 32/24 kg)

- 15 Kettlebell Goblet Squats (7(70/53 lbs - 32/24 kg)

- 10 Kettlebell Turkish Get-ups (5 each arm) (70/53 lbs - 32/24 kg) – scale down if needed

Vortex 5 Rounds for Time:

- 15 Kettlebell Swings (53/35 lbs - 24/16 kg)

- 15 Kettlebell Sumo Deadlift High Pulls (53/35 lbs - 24/16 kg)

- 200 meter Run

Whirlwind AMRAP in 15 minutes:

- 5 Kettlebell Turkish Get-ups (53/35 lbs - 24/16 kg)

- 10 Kettlebell Snatches (53/35 lbs - 24/16 kg)

- 15 Kettlebell Goblet Squats (53/35 lbs - 24/16 kg)

Zephyr For Time:

- 100 Kettlebell Swings (53/35 lbs - 24/16 kg)

- Every minute on the minute, perform 5 Burpees

Cyclone Challenge 5 Rounds for Time:

- 10 Kettlebell Windmills (35/22 lbs - 16/10 kg)

- 15 Kettlebell Swings (53/35 lbs - 24/16 kg)

- 200 meter Run

Dragon's Breath AMRAP in 15 minutes:

- 7 Kettlebell Snatches (53/35 lbs - 24/16 kg)

- 14 Kettlebell Goblet Squats (53/35 lbs - 24/16 kg)

- 21 Double-unders

Eagle's Nest 3 Rounds for Time:

- 20 Kettlebell Swings (70/53 lbs - 32/24 kg)

- 15 Kettlebell Deadlifts (70/53 lbs - 32/24 kg)

- 10 Kettlebell Turkish Get-ups (70/53 lbs - 32/24 kg)

Forge Fire For Time:

- 100 Kettlebell Thrusters (53/35 lbs - 24/16 kg)

- Every minute on the minute, perform 5 Kettlebell Swings (53/35 lbs - 24/16 kg)

Granite Grind 5 Rounds for Time:

- 10 Kettlebell Clean and Press (53/35 lbs - 24/16 kg)

- 20 Kettlebell Swings (53/35 lbs - 24/16 kg)

Hearthstone AMRAP in 12 minutes:

- 10 Kettlebell Snatches (53/35 lbs - 24/16 kg)

- 20 Kettlebell Goblet Squats (53/35 lbs - 24/16 kg)

- 30 Double Unders

Ivy League 4 Rounds for Time:

- 25 Kettlebell Swings (53/35 lbs - 24/16 kg)

- 50 Double Unders

Jade Mountain For Time:

- 100 Kettlebell Swings (53/35 lbs - 24/16 kg)

- Every minute on the minute, perform 5 Burpees

Keystone 10 Rounds for Time:

- 20 Kettlebell Clean and Jerks (35/22 lbs - 16/10 kg)

- 15 Kettlebell Goblet Squats (35/22 lbs - 16/10 kg)

- 10 Kettlebell Snatches (35/22 lbs - 16/10 kg)

Lion's Roar For Time:

- 50 Kettlebell Clean and Press (53/35 lbs - 24/16 kg)

- Every minute on the minute, perform 5 Box Jumps (24/20")

Monolit AMRAP in 20 minutes:

- 10 Kettlebell Swings (70/53 lbs - 32/24 kg)

- 20 Kettlebell Goblet Lunges (70/53 lbs - 32/24 kg)

- 30 Wall Balls (20/14 lbs - 9/6 kg)

- Rest 1 minute

Nexus Point 5 Rounds for Time:

- 20 Kettlebell Deadlifts(70/53 lbs - 32/24 kg)

- 15 Kettlebell Swings (70/53 lbs - 32/24 kg)

- 10 Kettlebell Thrusters (70/53 lbs - 32/24 kg)

Xenolith Xercise 4 Rounds for Time:

- 10 Kettlebell Turkish Get-ups (53/35 lbs - 24/16 kg)

- 20 Kettlebell Swings (53/35 lbs - 24/16 kg)

Yankee Doodle 5 Rounds for Time:

- 20 Kettlebell Deadlifts (70/53 lbs - 32/24 kg)

- 15 Kettlebell Swings (70/53 lbs - 32/24 kg)

- 10 Kettlebell Thrusters (70/53 lbs - 32/24 kg)

Oracle's Wisdom 4 Rounds for Time:

- 10 Kettlebell Turkish Get-ups (53/35 lbs - 24/16 kg)

- 20 Kettlebell Swings (53/35 lbs - 24/16 kg)

Pyramid Peak AMRAP in 15 minutes:

- 5 Kettlebell Snatches (70/53 lbs - 32/24 kg)

- 10 Kettlebell Clean and Jerks (70/53 lbs - 32/24 kg)

- 15 Kettlebell Goblet Squats (70/53 lbs - 32/24 kg)

Quartz Quest 4 Rounds for Time:

- 10 Kettlebell Snatches (53/35 lbs - 24/16 kg)

- 20 Kettlebell Swings (53/35 lbs - 24/16 kg)

- 30 Double Unders

River Run AMRAP in 20 minutes:

- 15 Kettlebell Swings (70/53 lbs - 32/24 kg)

- 30 Kettlebell Goblet Squats (70/53 lbs - 32/24 kg)

- 45 Double Unders

Steel Forge 5 Rounds for Time:

- 10 Kettlebell Deadlifts (70/53 lbs - 32/24 kg)

- 15 Kettlebell Swings (70/53 lbs - 32/24 kg)

- 20 Kettlebell Goblet Squats (70/53 lbs - 32/24 kg)

Titan's Strength For Time:

- 100 Kettlebell Thrusters (53/35 lbs - 24/16 kg)

- Every minute on the minute, perform 5 Kettlebell Swings (53/35 lbs - 24/16 kg)

Unbroken Chain 3 Rounds for Time:

- 20 Kettlebell Clean and Jerks (35/22 lbs - 16/10 kg)

- 15 Kettlebell Goblet Squats (35/22 lbs - 16/10 kg)

- 10 Kettlebell Snatches (35/22 lbs - 16/10 kg)

Valiant Vanguard For Time:

- 150 Kettlebell Snatches (53/35 lbs - 24/16 kg)

- Every minute on the minute, perform 5 Burpees

Warrior's Path AMRAP in 12 minutes:

- 10 Kettlebell Swings (53/35 lbs - 24/16 kg)

- 20 Kettlebell Goblet Squats (53 lbs / ~24 kg)

- 30 Double Unders

Zephyr's Speed AMRAP in 15 minutes:

- 5 Kettlebell Snatches (70/53 lbs - 32/24 kg)

- 10 Kettlebell Clean and Jerks (70/53 lbs - 32/24 kg)

- 15 Kettlebell Goblet Squats (70/53 lbs - 32/24 kg)

JUMP ROPE WORKOUTS

Jumping rope is more than a childhood pastime. It's an essential tool in the CrossFit arsenal, combining cardio, agility, and coordination in one simple, portable piece of equipment. Jump rope workouts can be as challenging as you want them to be, making them versatile and scalable for any fitness level.

In this chapter, we'll explore various jump rope workouts, from short and intense metcons to longer endurance sessions. The beauty of these workouts lies in their simplicity. You can perform them anywhere, making them ideal for home workouts or when you're traveling and have limited equipment.

Jump ropes are great for improving your footwork, speed, and timing - skills that transfer over to many other athletic endeavors. Additionally, they're a fantastic tool for fat burning and cardiovascular health.

Most of these workouts will incorporate the basic single-under and the more challenging double-under, where the rope passes under your feet twice per jump. We'll also include workouts that blend jump rope with other movements for a full-body workout.

As always, remember to prioritize good form, especially when fatigue sets in. Take care of your jump rope, and it will take care of you.

So, grab your rope, find some open space, and let's jump into it!

Double Twist For time:

- 150 Double Unders

- 50 Sit-Ups

- 100 Double Unders

- 50 Sit-Ups

- 50 Double Unders

- 50 Sit-Ups

Skipping Thunder 5 Rounds for time:

- 30 Single Unders

- 20 Air Squats

- 10 Push-ups

Rope Burn AMRAP in 12 minutes:

- 50 Double Unders

- 10 Burpees

Jumping Jack Flash 4 Rounds for time:

- 100 Single Unders

- 25 Jumping Jacks

- 50 Double Unders

- 25 Jumping Jacks

Crossrope Classic For time:

- 100 Double Unders

- 75 Air Squats

- 50 Push-ups

- 25 Pull-ups

- 100 Double Unders

Rope Climb Combo 3 Rounds for time:

- 30 Double Unders

- 3 Rope Climbs

- 30 Sit-ups

Heartbeat Skipper For time:

- 200 Single Unders

- 50 Sit-ups

- 40 Double Unders

- 20 Push-ups

- 20 Double Unders

- 10 Burpees

Bounce House AMRAP in 15 minutes:

- 100 Single Unders

- 20 Dumbbell Snatches (50/35 lbs - 23/16 kg)

- 10 Box Jumps (24/20")

Rhythm Runner 4 Rounds for time:

- 400 meter Run

- 100 Single Unders

Double-Double Dare For time:

- 100 Double Unders

- 50 Air Squats

- 100 Double Unders

- 50 Push-ups

- 100 Double Unders

- 50 Sit-ups

- 100 Double Unders

Cross Skipper 3 Rounds for time:

- 100 Double Unders

- 20 Lunges

- 10 Push-ups

Skipping Stones AMRAP in 12 minutes:

- 75 Double Unders

- 25 Air Squats

- 15 Push-ups

Rope 'n' Run For time:

- 400 meter Run

- 50 Double Unders

- 20 Sit-ups

- 10 Pull-ups

Jumprope Jamboree 4 Rounds for time:

- 50 Double Unders

- 25 Sit-ups

- 15 Air Squats

- 5 Push-ups

Rapid Ropes For time:

- 150 Double Unders

- 50 Air Squats

- 100 Double Unders

- 40 Push-ups

- 50 Double Unders

- 30 Sit-ups

Hopscotch Hero AMRAP in 15 minutes:

- 200 Single Unders

- 20 Box Jumps (24/20")

- 10 Pull-ups

Jumping Bean 5 Rounds for time:

- 50 Double Unders

- 10 Burpees

Twisted Rope 4 Rounds for time:

- 100 Single Unders

- 20 Lunges

- 10 Push-ups

Rope and Road For time:

- 800 meter Run

- 100 Double Unders

- 50 Sit-ups

Double Dutch AMRAP in 10 minutes:

- 50 Double Unders

- 10 Burpees

- 20 Sit-ups

Leaping Lizard For time:

- 100 Double Unders

- 50 Air Squats

- 100 Double Unders

- 40 Push-ups

- 100 Double Unders

- 30 Sit-ups

- 100 Double Unders

- 20 Burpees

- 100 Double Unders

- 10 Pull-ups

Jumping Jacks AMRAP in 15 minutes:

- 50 Double Unders

- 20 Walking Lunges

- 10 Push-ups

Rope and Run For time:

- 1 mile Run

- 100 Double Unders

- 800 meter Run

- 80 Double Unders

- 400 meter Run

- 60 Double Unders

- 200 meter Run

- 40 Double Unders

Skip to the Beat 5 Rounds for time:

- 50 Double Unders

- 10 Burpees

- 15 Sit-ups

Jumpstart 3 Rounds for time:

- 200 Single Unders

- 15 Box Jumps (24/20")

- 10 Pull-ups

Rope Burn AMRAP in 12 minutes:

- 100 Double Unders

- 15 Air Squats

- 10 Push-ups

Hop and Drop For time:

- 150 Double Unders

- 50 Air Squats

- 100 Double Unders

- 40 Push-ups

- 50 Double Unders

- 30 Sit-ups

Twist and Shout 5 Rounds for time:

- 50 Double Unders

- 20 Lunges

- 10 Push-ups

Rope Rumble 4 Rounds for time:

- 75 Single Unders

- 15 Wall Balls (20/14 lbs - 9/6 kg)

- 10 Pull-ups

Double Trouble AMRAP in 10 minutes:

- 100 Double Unders

- 10 Burpees

- 20 GHD Sit-ups

GYMNASTICS WORKOUTS

CrossFit is well-known for its integration of various fitness disciplines, and gymnastics is one of the core pillars that hold up the functional fitness roof. The body control, strength, flexibility, and balance developed through gymnastics movements are unparalleled and contribute significantly to overall fitness and athletic performance.

In this chapter, we delve into Gymnastics Workouts that solely or predominantly incorporate gymnastics movements. These exercises often use one's body weight as the primary resistance and demand a great deal of skill, coordination, and body awareness.

From pull-ups and push-ups to more advanced movements like muscle-ups, handstand push-ups, and pistols, these workouts will challenge you in unique ways. They'll improve your motor control, enhance your agility, and significantly contribute to your strength.

While these workouts might be challenging, particularly for those new to these movements, remember that every exercise can be scaled or modified. We'll discuss this more in our Scaling Options chapter.

Now, let's embrace the grace and grit of gymnastics with these workouts. On to the mat!

Practiced Poise 5 Rounds for Time:

- 10 Handstand Push-Ups

- 15 Toes-To-Bars

- 20 Box Jumps (24/20")

Frontline Flips 4 Rounds for Time:

- 50 Double-Unders

- 15 Ring Dips

- 10 Strict Pull-Ups

Vaulting Viper AMRAP in 15 Minutes:

- 5 Ring Muscle Ups

- 10 Pistol Squats (Alternating Legs)

- 15 GHD Sit-Ups

Balancing Bear For Time:

- 100 Double Unders

- 50 Handstand Push-Ups

- 100 Double Unders

- 50 Toes-to-Bars

- 100 Double Unders

Parallel Prowess 3 Rounds for Time:

- 20 Parallel Bar Handstand Push-Ups

- 30 Chest-to-Bar Pull-Ups

- 40 Alternating Pistol Squats

Springboard Swoop For Time:

- 50 Hand Release Push-Ups

- 40 Chest-to-Bar Pull-Ups

- 30 Handstand Push-Ups

- 20 Bar Muscle-Ups

- 10 Strict Ring Muscle-Ups

Tumbling Tiger AMRAP in 20 minutes:

- 5 Strict Handstand Push-Ups

- 10 Chest-to-Bar Pull-Ups

- 15 Toes-to-Bars

Rings of Resolve For Time:

- 30 Ring Muscle-Ups

- 60 Handstand Push-Ups

- 90 Toes-to-Bars

Gymnastic Gallop 5 Rounds for Time:

- 20 Double Unders
- 15 GHD Sit-Ups
- 10 Handstand Push-Ups
- 5 Strict Pull-Ups

Inverted Integrity 4 Rounds for Time:

- 25 Handstand Push-Ups
- 50 Double Unders
- 75 Air Squats

Undulating Unicorn For Time:

- 100 Air Squats
- 90 Sit-Ups
- 80 Alternating Lunges
- 70 Burpees
- 60-second Handstand Hold
- 50 Push-Ups
- 40 Hollow Rocks
- 30 Handstand Push-Ups
- 20 V-Ups

- 10 Strict Pull-Ups

Gymnast's Gauntlet 3 Rounds for Time:

- 10 Ring Muscle-Ups

- 20 Handstand Push-Ups

- 30 Pistols (Alternating Legs)

- 40 Double Unders

Lever Lift AMRAP in 15 Minutes:

- 5 Front Levers

- 10 Strict Toes-To-Bars

- 15 L-Sit Pull-Ups

Pommel Pace For Time:

- 75 Hollow Rocks

- 50 Handstand Push-Ups

- 25 Bar Muscle-Ups

Handspring Hustle AMRAP in 20 Minutes:

- 15 Handstand Push-Ups

- 20 Pistols (Alternating Legs)

- 25 Toes-to-Bars

Parallel Power 3 Rounds for Time:

- 10 Strict Handstand Push-Ups

- 15 Strict Pull-Ups

- 20 Pistols (Alternating Legs)

Beam Balance For Time:

- 50 Toes-to-Bars

- 40 Handstand Push-Ups

- 30 Ring Muscle-Ups

- 20 Pistol Squats (Alternating Legs)

- 10 Strict Handstand Push-Ups

Flipping Finch 4 Rounds for Time:

- 5 Strict Ring Muscle-Ups

- 10 Handstand Push-Ups

- 15 Toes-to-Bars

L-Sit Lark 5 Rounds for Time:

- 20 L-Sit Pull-Ups

- 30 Push-Ups

- 40 Air Squats

Cartwheeling Cougar For Time:

- 100 Double Unders

- 80 Air Squats

- 60 Push-Ups

- 40 Handstand Push-Ups

- 20 Bar Muscle-Ups

- 10 Front Levers

Rings of Saturn 4 Rounds for Time:

- 10 Strict Ring Dips

- 15 Toes-to-Bars

- 20 Alternating Pistols

Gymnast's Grind For Time:

- 50 Handstand Push-Ups

- 100 Hollow Rocks

- 150 Air Squats

Balance Beam Blitz 5 Rounds for Time:

- 5 Strict Handstand Push-Ups

- 10 L-Pull-Ups

- 15 Pistols (Alternating Legs)

Parallel Bars Push 3 Rounds for Time:

- 10 L-Sit Pull-Ups

- 20 Handstand Push-Ups

- 30 Air Squats

Handspring Hustle AMRAP in 20 Minutes:

- 10 Toes-to-Bars

- 20 Alternating Pistols

- 30 Double Unders

Uneven Bars Unleashed For Time:

- 30 Ring Muscle-Ups

- 60 Handstand Push-Ups

- 90 Air Squats

Mat Maneuvers 3 Rounds for Time:

- 20 Toes-to-Bars

- 40 Handstand Push-Ups

- 60 Double Unders

Grip and Grin For Time:

- 50 Strict Pull-Ups

- 100 Push-Ups

- 150 Air Squats

Pommel Horse Power 5 Rounds for Time:

- 10 Handstand Push-Ups

- 20 Toes-to-Bars

- 30 Double Unders

Vault Velocity AMRAP in 15 Minutes:

- 5 Strict Ring Muscle-Ups

- 10 Handstand Push-Ups

- 15 Pistols (Alternating Legs)

Strength Workouts

One of the foundational elements of CrossFit is strength training. In this chapter, we delve into workouts that prioritize building strength. Whether it's through classic barbell lifts, kettlebell work, or bodyweight movements, these workouts are designed to push your muscles to their limits and beyond.

In CrossFit, strength isn't just about raw power—it's about functional fitness. The aim is to cultivate strength that supports complex movements, overall physical health, and practical, everyday tasks. Strength workouts not only contribute to increased muscle mass and enhanced physical aesthetics, but they also play a crucial role in preventing injury, improving posture, boosting metabolic rate, and promoting better body mechanics.

From deadlifts to squats, snatches to clean and jerks, the workouts in this chapter will challenge both your maximal and submaximal strength. They will test and enhance your ability to express power through a range of movements and time domains.

Remember, it's essential to use correct technique when performing these strength workouts to avoid injury and maximize effectiveness. Always prioritize quality of movement over the weight lifted.

In the following section, you will find a collection of strength-focused workouts. These are designed to be integrated into your training program to develop and enhance your strength as part of a balanced fitness regimen. Let's lift!

Iron Forge For time:

- 10-9-8-7-6-5-4-3-2-1 Reps of:

- Deadlifts (225/155 lbs - 102/70 kg)

- Bench Press (135/96 lbs - 61/43 kg)

Steel Thunder 5 Rounds for time:

- 5 Overhead Squats (135/96 lbs - 61/43 kg)

- 10 Power Cleans (135/96 lbs - 61/43 kg)

- 15 Pull-Ups

Heavy Rain For time:

- 50 Back Squats (Bodyweight)

Boulder Dash 5 Rounds for time:

- 10 Front Squats (155/110 lbs - 70/50 kg)

- 10 Strict Handstand Push-ups

Titan Clash 3 Rounds for time:

- 5 Clean and Jerks (185/132 lbs - 84/60 kg)

- 10 Toes-to-Bar

Goliath's Fall For time:

- 100 Deadlifts (Bodyweight)

- Every minute on the minute, perform 5 burpees

Quartz Crumble 5 Rounds for time:

- 7 Thrusters (135/96 lbs - 61/43 kg)

- 14 Kettlebell Swings (70/53 lbs - 32/24 kg)

Granite Grind 3 Rounds for time:

- 10 Overhead Squats (135/96 lbs - 61/43 kg)

- 20 Pull-Ups

Sledgehammer Slam 4 Rounds for time:

- 8 Push Press (135/96 lbs - 61/43 kg)

- 12 Box Jumps (24/20")

Pyrite Crush 5 Rounds for time:

- 5 Deadlifts (225/155 lbs - 102/70 kg)

- 10 Burpees Over the Bar

Ferrum Force 3 Rounds for time:

- 10 Clean and Jerks (135/96 lbs - 61/43 kg)

- 20 Double Unders

Marble Breaker 4 Rounds for time:

- 12 Front Squats (155/110 lbs - 70/50 kg)

- 12 Toes-to-Bar

Platinum Pulse 5 Rounds for time:

- 10 Thrusters (95/65 lbs - 43/30 kg)

- 15 Pull-Ups

Quicksilver Quake 3 Rounds for time:

- 10 Snatches (115/81 lbs - 52/37 kg)

- 20 Box Jumps (24/20")

Rockslide Rumble 5 Rounds for time:

- 5 Overhead Squats (135/96 lbs - 61/43 kg)

- 10 Power Cleans (135/96 lbs - 61/43 kg)

Titanium Tumble For time:

- 100 Deadlifts (Bodyweight)

- Every minute on the minute, perform 3 Devil Press (2x 50/35 lbs - 23/16 kg)

Uranium Uproar 5 Rounds for time:

- 10 Push Press (135/96 lbs - 61/43 kg)

- 20 Kettlebell Swings (70/53 lbs - 32/24 kg)

Vulcan Vortex 3 Rounds for time:

- 10 Front Squats (155/110 lbs - 70/50 kg)

- 20 Strict Toes-to-Bar or Knee Raises

Zircon Zephyr 4 Rounds for time:

- 8 Clean and Jerks (135/96 lbs - 61/43 kg)

- 12 Box Jumps (24/20")

Argon Assault 3 Rounds for time:

- 10 Snatches (115/81 lbs - 52/37 kg)

- 20 Weighted Double Unders

Basalt Blast 5 Rounds for time:

- 5 Overhead Squats (135/96 lbs - 61/43 kg)

- 10 Power Cleans (135/96 lbs - 61/43 kg)

Cobalt Crush For time:

- 50 Back Squats (Bodyweight)

- Every minute on the minute, perform 5 burpees

Diamond Dust 5 Rounds for time:

- 10 Thrusters (95/65 lbs - 43/30 kg)

- 15 Pull-Ups

Emerald Eruption 3 Rounds for time:

- 10 Clean and Jerks (135/96 lbs - 61/43 kg)

- 20 Box Jumps (24/20")

Flint Flash 5 Rounds for time:

- 5 Deadlifts (225/155 lbs - 102/70 kg)

- 10 Burpees Over the Bar

Garnet Gale 3 Rounds for time:

- 10 Snatches (115/81 lbs - 52/37 kg)

- 20 Double Unders

Helium Heave 5 Rounds for time:

- 10 Push Press (135/96 lbs - 61/43 kg)

- 20 Kettlebell Swings (70/53 lbs - 32/24 kg)

Igneous Impact 3 Rounds for time:

- 10 Front Squats (155/110 lbs - 70/50 kg)

- 20 Toes-to-Bar

Jasper Jolt 4 Rounds for time:

- 8 Clean and Jerks (135/96 lbs - 61/43 kg)

- 12 Box Jumps (24/20")

Iron Climb 5 Rounds for Time:

- 5 Clean and Jerks (155/110 lbs - 70/50 kg)

- 10 Deadlifts (155/110 lbs - 70/50 kg)

- 15 Push-Ups

Steel Stomp AMRAP in 20 minutes:

- 5 Back Squats (185/132 lbs - 84/60 kg)

- 10 Kettlebell Swings (70/53 lbs - 32/24 kg)

- 15 Double-Unders

Titanium Push 4 Rounds for Time:

- 5 Overhead Squats (135/96 lbs - 61/43 kg)

- 10 Pull-ups

- 15 Sit-ups

Copper Charge For Time:

- 100 Dumbbell Thrusters (2x 50/35 lbs - 23/16 kg)

Alloy Ascend 5 Rounds for Time:

- 5 Snatches (115/81 lbs - 52/37 kg)

- 10 Toes-to-Bar

- 200 meter Run

Bronze Burn AMRAP in 12 minutes:

- 3 Front Squats (185/132 lbs - 84/60 kg)

- 6 Chest-to-Bar Pull-ups

- 9 Burpees

Platinum Punch 5 Rounds for Time:

- 7 Power Cleans (155/110 lbs - 70/50 kg)

- 14 Wall Balls (20/14 lbs - 9/6 kg)

Zinc Zest 3 Rounds for Time:

- 10 Deadlifts (225/155 lbs - 102/70 kg)

- 20 Push-ups

- 30 Double-Unders

Nickel Nudge For Time:

- 50 Push Presses (95/65 lbs - 43/30 kg)

- 100 Sit-ups

- 150 Double-Unders

Pewter Power AMRAP in 15 minutes:

- 5 Power Snatches (135/96 lbs - 61/43 kg)

- 10 Box Jumps (24/20")

Manganese Move 4 Rounds for Time:

- 10 Front Squats (155/110 lbs - 70/50 kg)

- 15 Kettlebell Swings (53/35 lbs - 24/16 kg)

- 200 meter Run

Silver Sprint For Time:

- 21 Overhead Squats (95/65 lbs - 43/30 kg)

- 42 Pull-ups

- 15 Overhead Squats (95/65 lbs - 43/30 kg)

- 30 Pull-ups

- 9 Overhead Squats (95/65 lbs - 43/30 kg)

- 18 Pull-ups

Gold Grind AMRAP in 20 minutes:

- 5 Power Cleans (155/110 lbs - 70/50 kg)

- 10 Toes-to-Bar

- 15 Wall Balls (20/14 lbs - 9/6 kg)

Chromium Chase 3 Rounds for Time:

- 10 Deadlifts (295/220 lbs - 134/100 kg)

- 20 Push-ups

- 30 Sit-ups

Titan Turmoil For Time:

- 100 Thrusters (45/33 lbs - 20/15 kg)

Cobalt Clash 5 Rounds for Time:

- 5 Snatches (135/96 lbs - 61/43 kg)

- 10 Pull-ups

- 200 meter Run

Lead Leap AMRAP in 12 minutes:

- 3 Front Squats (185/132 lbs - 84/60 kg)

- 6 Chest-to-Bar Pull-ups

- 9 Box Jumps (24/20")

Bismuth Burst 5 Rounds for Time:

- 7 Power Cleans (155/110 lbs - 70/50 kg)

- 14 Kettlebell Swings (53/35 lbs - 24/16 kg)

WEIGHTLIFTING TECHNIQUE WORKOUTS

Weightlifting is a critical component of CrossFit, requiring strength, power, mobility, and technique. In fact, many of the most challenging movements in CrossFit come from the Olympic weightlifting discipline, including the clean and jerk and the snatch. These movements are complex, requiring precision, coordination, and a strong understanding of body mechanics.

To master these skills, weightlifting technique workouts are indispensable. These workouts are designed to improve your form and efficiency, rather than aiming for maximum weight or speed. By emphasizing quality of movement over quantity of weight, you can reduce your risk of injury, improve your performance, and get more benefits out of your regular training.

During these workouts, the weight you choose to use should allow you to perform each rep with

perfect form. This might mean using a lighter weight than you would in a workout where you're aiming for a personal record. The goal is to practice the movement patterns, build muscle memory, and strengthen the specific muscles you'll use when lifting heavier weights. With this being said, we have provided a rough percentage for each workout which should be based from your 1 rep max of the movement.

Remember, these workouts are not about testing your limits, but rather about refining your technique. Over time, as your technique improves, you'll find that you can lift heavier weights more efficiently and safely. After all, the goal is not just to lift heavy, but to lift heavy well. Now, let's explore some weightlifting technique workouts to help you hone your craft.

Clean Catalyst (60%) EMOM for 15 minutes:

- 3 Power Cleans

- 3 Front Squats

- 3 Push Press

Deadlift Drill (80%) Five rounds for quality:

- 10 Romanian Deadlifts

- 10 Sumo Deadlifts

Jerk Jive (70%) Four rounds for quality:

- 5 Push Jerks

- 5 Split Jerks

- Rest 1 minute between rounds

Overhead Odyssey (90%) EMOM for 12 minutes:

- 2 Overhead Squats

Pull Power (85%) Five rounds for quality:

- 10 Power Snatches

- Rest 1 minute between rounds

Snatch Skill (70%) Four rounds for quality:

- 5 Power Snatches

- 5 Overhead Squats

Squat Sequence (75%) Five rounds for quality:

- 5 Front Squats

- 5 Back Squats

Thrust for Technique (60%) Four rounds for quality:

- 7 Thrusters

- Rest 1 minute between rounds

Unbroken Barbell (70%) AMRAP in 10 minutes:

- 5 Clean and Jerks

- 5 Snatches

Weightlifting Wisdom (90%) EMOM for 20 minutes:

- 1 Clean

- 1 Front Squat

- 1 Jerk

Bear Complex Bonanza (40%) Five rounds for quality:

- 7 Bear Complexes (Power Clean, Front Squat, Push Press, Back Squat, Push Press)

Clean and Jerk Journey (85%) EMOM for 20 minutes:

- 2 Clean and Jerks

Front Squat Focus (80%) Five rounds for quality:

- 5 Front Squats with 3-second pause at the bottom

Graceful Grip (50%) Four rounds for quality:

- 10 Hang Power Cleans

- 10 Hang Power Snatches

Overhead Stabilizer (80%) Four rounds for quality:

- 5 Overhead Squats with a 3-second pause at the bottom

Press Progression (60%) Four rounds for quality:

- 5 Push Presses

- 5 Push Jerks

Snatch Success (90%) EMOM for 15 minutes:

- 1 Snatches

Squat Clean Cycle (70%) Five rounds for quality:

- 5 Squat Cleans

Technique Triumph (70%) Four rounds for quality:

- 5 Snatches

- 5 Clean and Jerks

Thruster Therapy (50%) Five rounds for quality:

- 7 Thrusters

Under the Bar (110 – 120%) Four rounds for quality:

- 5 Clean Pulls

Overhead Stability (70%) Four rounds for quality:

- 5 Overhead Squats with a 2-second pause at the bottom

Power Hour (90%) EMOM for 15 minutes:

- 2 Power Cleans

Jerk Junction (75%) Five rounds for quality:

- 5 Split Jerks

Snatch Symphony (75%) Five rounds for quality:

- 5 Power Snatches

Clean Sweep (80%) Four rounds for quality:

- 5 Hang Squat Cleans

Pressing Matters (70%) Five rounds for quality:

- 5 Strict Presses

Lift-Off (95%) EMOM for 20 minutes:

- 1 Clean and Jerk

Front Squat Fortitude (80%) Four rounds for quality:

- 5 Front Squats with a 2-second pause at the bottom

Tempo Thruster Tune-Up (70%) Three rounds for quality:

- 7 Thrusters with a 3-second pause at the top

Deadlift Dance (95%) Four rounds for quality:

- 5 Deadlifts with a slow descent

Push Press Parade (70%) Five rounds for quality:

- 5 Push Presses with a controlled lowering phase

Snatch Cycle (60%) EMOM for 15 minutes:

- 2 Snatches with a pause at the knee

Clean Complex (70%) Four rounds for quality:

- 1 Power Clean + 1 Front Squat + 1 Hang Clean

Overhead Squat Symphony (60%) Four rounds for quality:

- 5 Overhead Squats with a pause at the bottom

Jerk Jamboree (70%) Five rounds for quality:

- 3 Split Jerks with a pause in the split

Lift Rhythm (75%) EMOM for 20 minutes:

- 1 Snatch + 1 Overhead Squat

Front Squat Fortitude (80%) Four rounds for quality:

- 5 Front Squats with a pause in the bottom and the halfway up position

Hang Clean Harmony (60%) Five rounds for quality:

- 5 Hang Cleans with a pause above the knee

ENDURANCE WORKOUTS

Endurance is a key aspect of fitness that CrossFit both tests and builds. This capacity to sustain prolonged physical or mental effort is crucial in many of the longer, more grueling workouts. Moreover, it's a fundamental element of overall health and wellbeing, impacting everything from cardiovascular health to mental resilience.

In CrossFit, endurance workouts typically involve sustained, lower-intensity efforts over a longer duration. These could range from longer runs, rows, or bike rides to workouts involving lighter weights and higher repetitions. The goal of these workouts is to challenge and expand your aerobic capacity and stamina, pushing your ability to maintain a steady pace over extended periods.

These workouts will test your mental toughness as much as your physical capabilities. As you fatigue, maintaining good form and a steady pace can become a challenge. Remember, it's not about how fast you start, but how well you can maintain your pace and your form as the workout progresses.

Endurance workouts can also provide a useful counterbalance to the heavier, more explosive workouts in your training. By incorporating both high-intensity and lower-intensity, longer-duration workouts into your routine, you can create a well-rounded fitness regimen that improves both your power and your stamina.

Ready to test your endurance? Let's dive into some endurance workouts that will challenge your staying power and help you build a solid aerobic base.

Stamina Surge 2 Rounds for Time:

- 2K Row

- 1K Run

Heartbeat Hustle 5 Rounds for Time:

- 400 meter Run

- 20 Box Step-ups

Endurance Elevation 3 Rounds for Time:

- 1K Row

- 50 Double Unders

- 1K Bike

Interval Ignition 8 Rounds, Each for Time:

- Run 400 meters

- Rest 1 minute

Quad Quell For Time:

- 10K Run

Breathe and Burn 5 Rounds for Time:

- Row 500 meters

- 15 Burpees

Oxygen Odyssey AMRAP in 35 minutes:

- 600 meter Run

- 20 Air Squats

Aerobic Ascension AMRAP in 30 minutes:

- Run 400 meters

- 30 Air Squats

- 30 Sit-ups

Resilience Rush 4 Rounds for Time:

- 400 meter Run

- 50 Double Unders

Longevity Leap For Time:

- 10K Row

Fuel the Fire AMRAP in 40 minutes:

- 800 meter Run

- 20 Walking Lunges

Gritty Grind For Time:

- 2K Row

- 1 mile Run

- 100 Double Unders

No Stopping Now For Time:

- 5K Bike

Mileage Mastery 3 Rounds for Time:

- 1 mile Bike

- 20 Burpees

Jog and Jump 4 Rounds for Time:

- 200 meter Run

- 50 Jump Ropes

Cardio Cascade 4 Rounds for Time:

- 800 meter Run

- 50 Jumping Jacks

Distance Divergence For Time:

- 5K Run

Tenacity Trail AMRAP in 40 minutes:

- 800 meter Run

- 20 Jumping Jacks

Pace Persistence 6 Rounds for Time:

- 500 meter Row

- Rest 2 minutes

Kilometer Cruise AMRAP in 45 minutes:

- 1K Run

- 20 Push-ups

Wind Sprint Wonders

4 Rounds for Time:

- Run 800 meters

- 25 Sit-ups

Mile Mover Three rounds for time:

- Run 1 mile

Sprint Specialist Eight rounds for time:

- 200 meter sprint

- Rest 2 minutes

Rowing Rumble For time:

- Row 5K

Double Under Dynamo For time:

- 1000 Double Unders

Trailblazer For time:

- Run 10K

Marathon Master For time:

- Run a Marathon (26.2 miles)

Ultra Undertaking For time:

- Run an Ultramarathon (50 miles)

Triathlon Triumph For time:

- 2.4 mile Swim

- 112 mile Bike

- 26.2 mile Run

Decathlon Dare Complete in any order:

- 100 meter Sprint

- 20 Broad Jumps

- 20 Wall Balls (20/14 lbs - 9/6 kg)

- 20 Burpees to Bar

- 400 meter Run

- 1500 meter Run

Pentathlon Pursuit Complete in order:

- 10 Wall Balls (20/14 lbs - 9/6 kg)

- 200 meter Run

- 20 Wall Balls (20/14 lbs - 9/6 kg)

- 400 meter Run

- 30 Wall Balls (20/14 lbs - 9/6 kg)

- 600 meter Run

- 40 Wall Balls (20/14 lbs - 9/6 kg)

- 800 meter Run

Olympic Odyssey For time:

- 1.5K Swim

- 40K Bike

- 10K Run

Half Ironman Hero For time:

- 1.2 mile Swim

- 56 mile Bike

- 13.1 mile Run

Ironman Icon For time:

- 2.4 mile Swim

- 112 mile Bike

- 26.2 mile Run

Cycling Century For time:

- Bike 100 miles

Dashing Decamile For time:

- Run 10 miles

Rowing Regatta For time:

- Row 10K

Swimathon Sensation For time:

- Swim 5K

Skiing Soiree For time:

- Ski 10K

RowErg Workouts

Welcome to the Row Erg Workouts chapter. Here, we shift our focus towards conditioning, stamina, and power, all through the versatility of the rowing machine or "Erg". The Row Erg is a staple of Cross-Fit and Cross Training regimes worldwide, providing a low-impact, high-intensity exercise that engages multiple muscle groups simultaneously.

A correctly used rowing machine can offer a comprehensive workout, targeting your legs, core, and upper body, all while improving your cardiovascular fitness. It is one of the few pieces of gym equipment that can claim to provide a full-body workout, and its benefits are numerous.

Rowing places equal emphasis on pushing and pulling movements, helping to balance the body's muscular development. Furthermore, the nature of rowing means that it can be tailored to specific workout goals: whether you're looking to improve your endurance, increase your power output, or simply to burn calories, the Row Erg can accommodate.

In this chapter, you'll find a selection of rowing workouts designed to challenge you and help you to improve your performance, whether you're a beginner, intermediate, or advanced athlete. For each workout, remember to focus on maintaining good form. The better your technique, the more effective your workout will be.

Let's get to it - the RowErg is waiting!

Rowing Rampage Workout Type: Long Distance
For time:

- Row 3000 meters

Pacing Information: Aim to maintain a steady pace throughout, with a split time of 2:00/500m.

Glacier Glide Workout Type: Medium Distance
For time:

- Row 2000 meters

Pacing Information: Aim for a steady 2:00/500m pace.

Maelstrom Madness Workout Type: Short Distance
For time:

- Row 500 meters

Pacing Information: Aim for a challenging, but manageable pace.

Crimson Cruise Workout Type: Long Distance
For time:

- Row 10,000 meters

Pacing Information: Maintain a consistent pace, targeting around 2:15/500m.

Riptide Rush Workout Type: Calories
For time:

- Burn 300 calories

Pacing Information: Aim for a consistent and sustainable pace.

Tidal Triumph Workout Type: Intervals
10 rounds of:

- Row 250 meters

- Rest 1 minute

Pacing Information: Push hard during the work periods, aim for 1:40/500m pace.

Ocean Odyssey Workout Type: Time
For time:

- Row for 30 minutes

Pacing Information: Try to maintain a consistent pace throughout.

Poseidon's Pulse Workout Type: Sprints
8 rounds of:

- Row 100 meters

- Rest 30 seconds

Pacing Information: Sprint during work periods, rest on the rest period.

Surfing the Surge Workout Type: Distance
For time:

- Row 5,000 meters

Pacing Information: Aim for a steady 2:05/500m pace.

Abyssal Ascend Workout Type: Long Distance
For time:

- Row 42,195 meters

Pacing Information: Maintain a consistent pace, targeting around 2:30/500m.

Wave Whisperer Workout Type: Intervals
5 rounds of:

- Row 500 meters

- Rest 2 minutes

Pacing Information: Push hard during the work periods, aim for 1:50/500m pace.

Neptune's Nudge Workout Type: Short Distance
For time:

- Row 1,000 meters

Pacing Information: Aim for a challenging, but manageable pace.

Pearl Plunge Workout Type: Time
For time:

- Row for 60 minutes

Pacing Information: Try to maintain a consistent pace throughout.

Coral Climb Workout Type: Intervals
4 rounds of:

- Row 750 meters

- Rest 1 minute

Pacing Information: Push hard during the work periods, aim for 1:45/500m pace.

Pelagic Pace Workout Type: Distance
For time:

- Row 3,000 meters

Pacing Information: Aim for a steady 2:00/500m pace.

Atlantis Amble Workout Type: Long Distance
For time:

- Row 21,097 meters

Pacing Information: Maintain a consistent pace, targeting around 2:20/500m.

Marine Marathon Workout Type: Time
For time:

- Row for 45 minutes

Pacing Information: Try to maintain a consistent pace throughout.

Siren Sprint Workout Type: Sprints
10 rounds of:

- Row 200 meters

- Rest 1 minute

Pacing Information: Sprint during work periods, rest on the rest period.

Nautical Navigate Workout Type: Calories
For time:

- Burn 200 calories

Pacing Information: Aim for a consistent and sustainable pace.

Current Challenge Workout Type: Intervals
3 rounds of:

- Row 1,000 meters

- Rest 2 minutes

Pacing Information: Push hard during the work periods, aim for 1:55/500m pace.

Tsunami Tempo Workout Type: Short Distance
For time:

- Row 750 meters

Pacing Information: Aim for a challenging, but manageable pace.

Vortex Voyage Workout Type: Medium Distance For time:

- Row 2,500 meters

Pacing Information: Aim for a steady 2:00/500m pace.

Whirlpool Wander Workout Type: Intervals
5 rounds of:

- Row 350 meters

- Rest 1 minute

Pacing Information: Push hard during the work periods, aim for 1:45/500m pace.

Depth Drive Workout Type: Long Distance
For time:

- Row 15,000 meters

Pacing Information: Maintain a consistent pace, targeting around 2:10/500m.

Mariner's Milestone Workout Type: Time
For time:

- Row for 40 minutes

Pacing Information: Try to maintain a consistent pace throughout.

Tide Tackle Workout Type: Sprints
6 rounds of:

- Row 150 meters

- Rest 30 seconds

Pacing Information: Sprint during work periods, rest on the rest period.

Fathom Flight Workout Type: Distance
For time:

- Row 4,000 meters

Pacing Information: Aim for a steady 2:05/500m pace.

Oceanic Orbit Workout Type: Calories
For time:

- Burn 250 calories

Pacing Information: Aim for a consistent and sustainable pace.

Seafarer's Stride Workout Type: Intervals
7 rounds of:

- Row 300 meters

- Rest 1 minute

Pacing Information: Push hard during the work periods, aim for 1:40/500m pace.

Harbor Hustle Workout Type: Short Distance
For time:

- Row 800 meters

Pacing Information: Aim for a challenging, but manageable pace.

Bayou Blitz Workout Type: Medium Distance
For time:

- Row 1,500 meters

Pacing Information: Aim for a steady 1:55/500m pace.

SkiErg Workouts

The SkiErg, an iconic piece of equipment found in many CrossFit and Cross Training gyms, offers a full-body, low-impact workout that effectively targets strength and endurance. It emulates the motion of cross-country skiing, a sport renowned for its high cardiovascular demands. Unlike traditional skiing, however, the SkiErg can be used year-round, regardless of weather conditions.

This equipment requires coordination of both the upper and lower body, engaging your core, arms, shoulders, and legs in a dynamic pulling motion. The SkiErg can also be used for both double pole and classic alternating arm technique. The workouts in this chapter will challenge your muscular and cardiovascular systems, improving your overall fitness, strength, and endurance. The versatility of the SkiErg makes it a valuable tool in any CrossFit or Cross Training regimen.

Alpine Ascend Workout Type: Long Distance
For time:

- Ski 10,000 meters

Pacing Information: Maintain a steady and sustainable pace throughout, focusing on form and rhythm.

Blizzard Beatdown Workout Type: Intervals
8 Rounds of:

- Ski 500 meters

- Rest 2 minutes

Pacing Information: Aim for high intensity during your skiing intervals, resting fully between sets.

Crystal Cruise Workout Type: Medium Distance
For time:

- Ski 5,000 meters

Pacing Information: Maintain a consistent rhythm and pace that allows you to finish without unnecessary breaks.

Downhill Dash Workout Type: Short Distance
For time:

- Ski 1,000 meters

Pacing Information: Push hard, this is a sprint. Aim to maintain a high intensity throughout.

Elevation Effort Workout Type: Calories
AMRAP in 20 minutes:

- Ski for Calories

Pacing Information: Try to find a sustainable, yet challenging pace that you can maintain for the whole 20 minutes.

Frosty Furlong Workout Type: Time
Ski as far as possible in:

- 30 minutes

Pacing Information: Maintain a steady pace that feels challenging but sustainable for the full 30 minutes.

Glacial Grind Workout Type: Intervals
10 Rounds of:

- Ski 200 meters

- Rest 1 minute

Pacing Information: Aim for a high intensity during your skiing intervals, resting fully between sets.

Horizon Hike Workout Type: Long Distance
For time:

- Ski 15,000 meters

Pacing Information: This is a long workout. Aim to maintain a steady, sustainable pace.

Icecapade Intensity Workout Type: Calories
For time:

- Ski 100 Calories

Pacing Information: Try to burn those calories as fast as possible. It's going to be intense!

Jubilant Journey Workout Type: Medium Distance
For time:

- Ski 7,500 meters

Pacing Information: Try to maintain a consistent pace throughout the workout, avoiding unnecessary breaks.

Kilometer Krusher Workout Type: Intervals
10 Rounds of:

- Ski 500 meters

- Rest 2 minutes

Pacing Information: Aim for a high intensity during your skiing intervals, resting fully between sets.

Lustrous Laps Workout Type: Time
Ski as far as possible in:

- 45 minutes

Pacing Information: Find a sustainable pace that allows you to ski for the entire duration without stopping.

Meteor Mile Workout Type: Short Distance
For time:

- Ski 1,600 meters

Pacing Information: Push hard, this is a sprint. Try to maintain a high intensity throughout.

Nordic Nightmare Workout Type: Calories
AMRAP in 30 minutes:

- Ski for Calories

Pacing Information: Find a rhythm that allows you to accumulate as many calories as possible.

Oblivion Orbit Workout Type: Long Distance
For time:

- Ski 10,000 meters

Pacing Information: This is a marathon, not a sprint. Find a sustainable pace and stick to it.

Polar Plunge Workout Type: Intervals
5 Rounds of:

- Ski 1,000 meters

- Rest 3 minutes

Pacing Information: Aim for a high intensity during your skiing intervals, resting fully between sets.

Quicksilver Quell Workout Type: Time
Ski as far as possible in:

- 60 minutes

Pacing Information: Try to maintain a steady pace that feels challenging but sustainable for the full hour.

Ridge Race Workout Type: Medium Distance
For time:

- Ski 6,000 meters

Pacing Information: Aim to maintain a consistent rhythm and pace that allows you to finish without unnecessary breaks.

Slope Sprint Workout Type: Short Distance
For time:

- Ski 500 meters

Pacing Information: This is a short, intense workout. Give it everything you've got!

Tundra Trek Workout Type: Calories
For time:

- Ski 200 Calories

Pacing Information: This will be tough. Push as hard as you can to burn those calories!

Uphill Undertaking Workout Type: Long Distance
For time:

- Ski 20,000 meters

Pacing Information: This is a long workout. Aim to maintain a steady, sustainable pace.

Vista Voyage Workout Type: Intervals
8 Rounds of:

- Ski 400 meters

- Rest 2 minutes

Pacing Information: Aim for a high intensity during your skiing intervals, resting fully between sets.

Winter Wander Workout Type: Medium Distance
For time:

- Ski 8,000 meters

Pacing Information: Try to maintain a consistent pace throughout the workout, avoiding unnecessary breaks.

Xtreme X-Country Workout Type: Time
Ski as far as possible in:

- 40 minutes

Pacing Information: Find a sustainable pace that allows you to ski for the entire duration without stopping.

Yonder Yomp Workout Type: Short Distance
For time:

- Ski 750 meters

Pacing Information: This is a sprint. Push hard and try to maintain a high intensity throughout.

Zenith Zoom Workout Type: Calories
AMRAP in 15 minutes:

- Ski for Calories

*Pacing Information: Find a rhythm that allows you to accumulate as many calories

BikeErg Workouts

The BikeErg, developed by the esteemed Concept2 creators, has quickly become a staple in the world of Cross Training and CrossFit. Despite its recent introduction, it's already made a name for itself as a rigorous and effective tool for cardiovascular training. Unlike traditional stationary or spin bikes, the BikeErg's design utilizes air resistance to create a smooth, stable ride that can be easily adjusted to meet the user's desired intensity.

While the BikeErg is an excellent tool for steady-state cardio and recovery rides, it also shines when incorporated into high-intensity workouts. This chapter will provide a range of BikeErg workouts that challenge your endurance, strength, and power. As always, remember to scale the workouts according to your fitness level and capabilities. In the case of the BikeErg, this could mean adjusting the damper setting, the workout duration, or the distance.

Now, let's get pedaling!

Cyclone Sprint *Workout Type: Distance*
5 Rounds for time:

- Sprint 500 meters on BikeErg

- Rest 2 minutes

Pacing Information: Aim to maintain a consistent pace across all rounds. Record your time for each round to track your consistency.

Endurance Hour *Workout Type: Time*
For time:

- 60 minutes of steady state biking on BikeErg

Pacing Information: Keep a consistent pace that feels challenging but sustainable for the full hour. This should be a pace at which you can maintain a conversation.

Calorie Crusher *Workout Type: Calories*
For time:

- Burn 200 calories on BikeErg

Pacing Information: Set a strong, sustainable pace from the beginning. Aim for consistent power output to steadily chip away at the calories.

Interval Ignition *Workout Type: Intervals*
10 Rounds for time:

- 1 minute of high-intensity biking on BikeErg

- 1 minute of rest

Pacing Information: During the high-intensity minute, aim to push your limits while maintaining a strong, steady cadence. Use the rest minute to recover.

Pace Perseverance *Workout Type: Pace*
4 Rounds for time:

- 10 minutes biking at a 75 RPM pace on BikeErg

- 2 minutes rest

Pacing Information: Try to maintain the 75 RPM pace throughout the 10 minutes of work. Use the rest time to recover and prepare for the next round.

Watt Wizard *Workout Type: Power (Watts)*
For time:

- 30 minutes biking on BikeErg at a target of 200 watts

Pacing Information: Try to maintain a consistent power output of 200 watts throughout the workout. This will require a balance of speed and resistance.

Torque Tenacity *Workout Type: Power (Watts)*
3 Rounds for time:

- 10 minutes biking at a target of 150 watts on BikeErg

- 2 minutes rest

Pacing Information: Aim to maintain a consistent power output of 150 watts throughout each round.

Calorie Clash *Workout Type: Calories*
AMRAP in 20 minutes:

- Burn as many calories as possible on BikeErg

Pacing Information: Pace yourself to sustain maximum effort for the full 20 minutes. Note total calories burned for tracking progress.

Stamina Surge *Workout Type: Time*
For time:

- 45 minutes of steady state biking on BikeErg

Pacing Information: Maintain a pace that allows for steady, continuous movement for the full 45 minutes.

Revolution Rampage *Workout Type: Intervals*
8 Rounds for time:

- 2 minutes of high-intensity biking on BikeErg

- 1 minute of rest

Pacing Information: Aim for a high RPM during the work periods. The goal is to maintain as high a cadence as possible for each 2-minute round.

Distance Dare *Workout Type: Distance*
For time:

- Bike 10,000 meters on BikeErg

Pacing Information: Set a challenging but sustainable pace that will allow you to continuously chip away at the distance.

Pace Persistence *Workout Type: Pace*
5 Rounds for time:

- 5 minutes biking at a 80 RPM pace on BikeErg

- 1 minute rest

Pacing Information: Try to maintain the 80 RPM pace throughout the 5 minutes of work. Use the rest time to recover and prepare for the next round.

Watt Warrior *Workout Type: Power (Watts)*
For time:

- 20 minutes biking on BikeErg at a target of 225 watts

Pacing Information: Try to maintain a consistent power output of 225 watts throughout the workout.

Calorie Conquest *Workout Type: Calories*
For time:

- Burn 500 calories on BikeErg

Pacing Information: Set a strong, sustainable pace from the beginning. Aim for consistent power output to steadily chip away at the calories.

Endurance Expedition *Workout Type: Time*
For time:

- 90 minutes of steady state biking on BikeErg

Pacing Information: Keep a consistent pace that feels challenging but sustainable for the full 90 minutes. This should be a pace at which you can maintain a conversation.

Interval Inferno *Workout Type: Intervals*
6 Rounds for time:

- 3 minute of high-intensity biking on BikeErg

- 2 minute of rest

Pacing Information: During the high-intensity minute, aim to push your limits while maintaining a strong, steady cadence. Use the rest minute to recover.

Pace Pursuit *Workout Type: Pace*
6 Rounds for time:

- 8 minutes biking at a 70 RPM pace on BikeErg

- 2 minutes rest

Pacing Information: Try to maintain the 70 RPM pace throughout the 8 minutes of work. Use the rest time to recover and prepare for the next round.

Watt Wonder *Workout Type: Power (Watts)*
For time:

- 25 minutes biking on BikeErg at a target of 250 watts

Pacing Information: Try to maintain a consistent power output of 250 watts throughout the workout.

Calorie Crusade *Workout Type: Calories*

For time:

- Burn 300 calories on BikeErg

Pacing Information: Set a strong, sustainable pace from the beginning. Aim for consistent power output to steadily chip away at the calories.

Stamina Sprint *Workout Type: Time*
For time:

- 30 minutes of steady state biking on BikeErg

Pacing Information: Maintain a pace that allows for steady, continuous movement for the full 30 minutes.

Revolution Rally *Workout Type: Intervals*
10 Rounds for time:

- 1 minute of high-intensity biking on BikeErg

- 1 minute of rest

Pacing Information: Aim for a high RPM during the work periods. The goal is to maintain as high a cadence as possible for each 1-minute round.

Distance Dash *Workout Type: Distance*
For time:

- Bike 5,000 meters on BikeErg

Pacing Information: Set a challenging but sustainable pace that will allow you to continuously chip away at the distance.

Pace Persistence *Workout Type: Pace*
4 Rounds for time:

- 10 minutes biking at a 85 RPM pace on BikeErg

- 2 minutes rest

Pacing Information: Try to maintain the 85 RPM pace throughout the 10 minutes of work. Use the rest time to recover and prepare for the next round.

Watt Wizard *Workout Type: Power (Watts)*
For time:

- 15 minutes biking on BikeErg at a target of 275 watts

Pacing Information: Try to maintain a consistent power output of 275 watts throughout the workout.

Calorie Challenge *Workout Type: Calories*
For time:

- Burn 100 calories on BikeErg

Pacing Information: Set a strong, sustainable pace from the beginning. Aim for consistent power output to steadily chip away at the calories.

Endurance Energy *Workout Type: Time*
For time:

- 75 minutes of steady state biking on BikeErg

Pacing Information: Keep a consistent pace that feels challenging but sustainable for the full 75 minutes.

ASSAULT BIKE OR ECOBIKE WORKOUTS

For any fitness enthusiast, Assault Bike or EcoBike workouts offer a unique challenge. Unlike other stationary bikes, these full-body cardiovascular machines engage both your upper and lower body, leading to a high calorie burn in a short amount of time. They are also known for their ability to ramp up the intensity quickly, making them an excellent tool for interval training. The resistance on these bikes is air-based; the harder you pedal, the more resistance you create, making the workout incredibly challenging and effective. Whether you're aiming to improve your endurance, burn fat, or enhance your athletic performance, these workouts can be a key part of your fitness routine.

From cycling for calories to pushing for time or distance, these workouts encompass a variety of training modalities, offering ample opportunity to challenge yourself in new and exciting ways. Regardless of your fitness level, these Assault Bike or EcoBike workouts can be scaled to meet you where you're at, making them an excellent addition to any fitness regimen. Let's dive in!

Calorie Crusher Workout Type: Calories
For time:

- Bike 30 calories

Pacing Information: This is a sprint, aim to burn through these calories as fast as possible.

Caloric Crusade Workout Type: Calories
For Time:

- Burn 100 calories

- Rest 2 minutes

- Burn 75 calories

- Rest 2 minutes

- Burn 50 calories

- Rest 2 minutes

- Burn 25 calories

Pacing Information: Start at a moderate pace for the 100 calories, then aim to increase your intensity as the calories decrease.

RPM Rumble Workout Type: RPM
EMOM for 20 minutes:

- 20 seconds at 70 RPM

- 40 seconds at 50 RPM

Pacing Information: Aim to maintain the RPM goals for each interval.

Wattage Wipeout Workout Type: Watts
5 Rounds:

- 1 minute at 200 Watts

- 1 minute rest

Pacing Information: Aim to maintain 200 Watts during the working minute. Use the rest minute to recover.

Distance Dilemma Workout Type: Distance
For Time:

- Bike 10 miles

Pacing Information: Aim to maintain a steady pace you can sustain for the full 10 miles.

Time Tracker Workout Type: Time
5 Rounds:

- 3 minutes of biking

- 2 minutes of rest

Pacing Information: Aim for a high, but sustainable pace during the 3 minutes of work.

Heart Rate Hustle Workout Type: Heart Rate
4 Rounds:

- 4 minutes at 80% max heart rate

- 3 minutes at 60% max heart rate

Pacing Information: Use a heart rate monitor to maintain the desired heart rate zones.

Wattage Wave Workout Type: Watts
10 Rounds:

- 30 seconds at 250 Watts

- 30 seconds at 150 Watts

Pacing Information: Aim to maintain the specified wattage for each interval.

Caloric Challenge Workout Type: Calories
For Time:

- Burn 50 calories at a slow pace

- Burn 50 calories at a moderate pace

- Burn 50 calories at a fast pace

Pacing Information: Increase your pace as you move through the calories.

Distance Dash Workout Type: Distance
3 Rounds for time:

- Bike 3 miles at a fast pace

- Bike 2 miles at a moderate pace

- Bike 1 mile at a slow pace

Pacing Information: Adjust your speed based on the distance for each interval.

Time Tussle Workout Type: Time
AMRAP in 20 minutes:

- 2 minutes at a fast pace

- 1 minute at a slow pace

Pacing Information: Alternate between a fast and slow pace every minute.

RPM Relay Workout Type: RPM
5 Rounds:

- 1 minute at 60 RPM

- 1 minute at 70 RPM

- 1 minute at 80 RPM

- 1 minute rest

Pacing Information: Increase your RPM with each minute, then recover during the rest minute.

Wattage Wonder Workout Type: Watts
4 Rounds:

- 2 minutes at 200 Watts

- 1 minute at 100 Watts

- 2 minutes rest

Pacing Information: Aim to maintain the specified wattage for each interval, then recover during the rest minutes.

Caloric Climb Workout Type: Calories
For Time:

- Burn 20 calories at a slow pace

- Burn 40 calories at a moderate pace

- Burn 60 calories at a fast pace

- Burn 40 calories at a moderate pace

- Burn 20 calories at a slow pace

Pacing Information: Adjust your pace as you move through the calories.

Distance Determination Workout Type: Distance
For Time:

- Bike 15 miles

Pacing Information: Aim to maintain a steady pace you can sustain for the full 15 miles.

Heart Rate Rampage Workout Type: Heart Rate
6 Rounds:

- 3 minutes at 70% max heart rate

- 2 minutes at 60% max heart rate

Pacing Information: Use a heart rate monitor to maintain the desired heart rate zones.

Time Torment Workout Type: Time
AMRAP in 30 minutes:

- 3 minutes at a fast pace

- 2 minutes at a moderate pace

- 1 minute at a slow pace

Pacing Information: Alternate between a fast, moderate, and slow pace every 6 minutes.

Wattage War Workout Type: Watts
8 Rounds:

- 30 seconds at 300 Watts

- 1 minute at 200 Watts

- 1 minute rest

Pacing Information: Aim to maintain the specified wattage for each interval, then recover during the rest minute.

Caloric Chaos Workout Type: Calories
For Time:

- Burn 75 calories at a fast pace

- Burn 50 calories at a moderate pace

- Burn 25 calories at a slow pace

Pacing Information: Decrease your pace as you move through the calories.

RPM Resilience Workout Type: RPM
4 Rounds:

- 1 minute at 75 RPM

- 2 minutes at 65 RPM

- 3 minutes at 55 RPM

- 2 minutes rest

Pacing Information: Decrease your RPM with each interval, then recover during the rest minutes.

Distance Defiance Workout Type: Distance
2 Rounds:

- Bike 5 miles at a fast pace

- Bike 5 miles at a moderate pace

- Bike 5 miles at a slow pace

Pacing Information: Adjust your speed based on the distance for each interval.

Wattage Whirlwind Workout Type: Watts
10 Rounds:

- 1 minute at 250 Watts

- 1 minute at 150 Watts

Pacing Information: Aim to maintain the specified wattage for each interval.

Heart Rate Heroics Workout Type: Heart Rate
4 Rounds:

- 4 minutes at 80% max heart rate

- 3 minutes at 60% max heart rate

- 2 minutes rest

Pacing Information: Use a heart rate monitor to maintain the desired heart rate zones.

Caloric Clash Workout Type: Calories
For Time:

- Burn 30 calories at a slow pace

- Burn 60 calories

at a moderate pace

- Burn 90 calories at a fast pace

Pacing Information: Increase your pace as you move through the calories.

RPM Rush Workout Type: RPM
EMOM for 30 minutes:

- 30 seconds at 80 RPM

- 30 seconds at 60 RPM

Pacing Information: Aim to maintain the RPM goals for each interval.

Time Turmoil Workout Type: Time
5 Rounds:

- 4 minutes of biking

- 1 minute of rest

Pacing Information: Aim for a high, but sustainable pace during the 4 minutes of work.

Distance Decathlon Workout Type: Distance
For Time:

- Bike 2 miles at a fast pace

- Bike 4 miles at a moderate pace

- Bike 6 miles at a slow pace

Pacing Information: Adjust your speed based on the distance for each interval.

Wattage Warfare Workout Type: Watts
6 Rounds:

- 2 minutes at 250 Watts

- 1 minute at 150 Watts

- 2 minutes rest

Pacing Information: Aim to maintain the specified wattage for each interval, then recover during the rest minutes.

Heart Rate Havoc Workout Type: Heart Rate
5 Rounds:

- 5 minutes at 70% max heart rate

- 3 minutes at 60% max heart rate

- 2 minutes rest

Pacing Information: Use a heart rate monitor to maintain the desired heart rate zones.

RUNNING WORKOUTS

Running has been a cornerstone of fitness for millennia, from the earliest hunter-gatherers to today's high-performance athletes. It's a fundamental movement, a full-body exercise, and a phenomenal way to develop cardiovascular endurance, speed, and agility. Whether you're pounding the pavement, hitting the trails, or striding on a treadmill, running is a versatile and accessible way to get fit and stay fit.

In this chapter, we'll explore a variety of running workouts designed to challenge your body and mind in different ways. We'll combine the simple act of running with the principles of Cross Training and CrossFit to create dynamic, high-intensity workouts that can help you reach your fitness goals. Whether you're a seasoned runner looking for a new challenge or a fitness enthusiast wanting to incorporate more running into your routine, you'll find workouts here to suit your needs.

Leapfrog Sprints Workout Type: Intervals
5 rounds:

- Sprint 200 meters

- Rest 1 minute

Pacing Information: Aim to run each sprint at 85-90% of your maximum effort. Focus on maintaining a fast and consistent pace for each sprint.

Tempo Tango Workout Type: Tempo Run
For time:

- Run 5 miles

Pacing Information: Run at a comfortably hard pace, about 75-80% of your maximum effort. Try to maintain a consistent pace throughout the entire run.

Hill Hunter Workout Type: Hill Repeats
8 rounds:

- Run uphill for 2 minutes

- Walk downhill to recover

Pacing Information: Push hard during the uphill sections, aiming for 80-85% of your maximum effort. Use the downhill walk to recover and prepare for the next uphill run.

Fartlek Frenzy Workout Type: Fartlek
For 30 minutes:

- Alternate between 2 minutes of easy running and 1 minute of fast running

Pacing Information: During the easy running segments, maintain a relaxed and comfortable pace. During the fast segments, aim for 85-90% of your maximum effort.

The Mile Crusher Workout Type: Time Trial
For time:

- Run 1 mile

Pacing Information: Aim to complete the mile as fast as possible, pushing yourself to maintain a high intensity throughout the run. This is a test of your speed and endurance.

Rising Sun Workout Type: Long Slow Distance
For time:

- Run 10 miles

Pacing Information: Run at a comfortable, conversational pace, about 60-70% of your maximum effort. Focus on maintaining a steady rhythm and staying relaxed throughout the run.

Ladder Speed Workout Type: Intervals
For time:

- Run 400 meters

- Rest 2 minutes

- Run 800 meters

- Rest 3 minutes

- Run 1200 meters

- Rest 4 minutes

- Run 800 meters

- Rest 3 minutes

- Run 400 meters

Pacing Information: Aim for a challenging pace during the running intervals, around 80-85% of your maximum effort. Use the rest periods to recover and prepare for the next interval.

Progressive Pacer Workout Type: Progression Run
For time:

- Run 6 miles, increasing pace every 2 miles

Pacing Information: Start at a comfortable, easy pace for the first 2 miles. Increase your pace to a moderately hard effort for the next 2 miles, and then finish the last 2 miles at a challenging, near-maximum effort.

Cadence Cadet Workout Type: Cadence Run
For 20 minutes:

- Focus on maintaining a cadence of 180 steps per minute

Pacing Information: Adjust your running speed to maintain the target cadence. This workout is designed to help improve running efficiency and form.

Rolling Relays Workout Type: Intervals
8 rounds:

- Run 400 meters

- Rest 1:1 (rest the same amount of time it took to complete the previous 400 meters)

Pacing Information: Aim to run each interval at a fast pace, around 85-90% of your maximum effort. Use the rest periods to recover and focus on maintaining a consistent pace for each interval.

Endless Endurance Workout Type: Long Slow Distance
For time:

- Run 15 miles

Pacing Information: Run at a comfortable, conversational pace, about 60-70% of your maximum effort. Focus on maintaining a steady rhythm and staying relaxed throughout the run.

Sprint Symphony Workout Type: Intervals
8 rounds:

- Sprint 100 meters

- Walk 100 meters

Pacing Information: Run each sprint at near-maximum effort. Use the walk back as your recovery period.

Marathon Mimic Workout Type: Long Distance
For time:

- Run 26.2 miles

Pacing Information: Aim to maintain a steady pace that feels challenging but sustainable for the full distance.

Quick Quarters Workout Type: Intervals
10 rounds:

- Run 400 meters

- Rest 2 minutes

Pacing Information: Aim to run each 400 meters at a fast, challenging pace. Use the 2-minute rest periods to recover.

Tempo Trailblazer Workout Type: Tempo Run
For time:

- Run 8 miles

Pacing Information: Run at a comfortably hard pace, about 75-80% of your maximum effort. Try to maintain a consistent pace throughout the entire run.

Hilltop Hustle Workout Type: Hill Repeats
6 rounds:

- Run uphill for 3 minutes

- Walk downhill to recover

Pacing Information: Push hard during the uphill sections, aiming for 80-85% of your maximum effort. Use the downhill walk to recover and prepare for the next uphill run.

Fartlek Fable Workout Type: Fartlek
For 45 minutes:

- Alternate between 3 minutes of easy running and 1 minute

of fast running

Pacing Information: During the easy running segments, maintain a relaxed and comfortable pace. During the fast segments, aim for 85-90% of your maximum effort.

Half-Marathon Harmony Workout Type: Long Distance
For time:

- Run 13.1 miles

Pacing Information: Aim to maintain a steady pace that feels challenging but sustainable for the full distance.

Ascending Agony Workout Type: Intervals
For time:

- Run 200 meters

- Rest 1 minute

- Run 400 meters

- Rest 2 minutes

- Run 800 meters

- Rest 4 minutes

- Run 1600 meters

Pacing Information: Aim for a challenging pace during the running intervals, around 80-85% of your maximum effort. Use the rest periods to recover and prepare for the next interval.

Progressive Pedestrian Workout Type: Progression Run
For time:

- Run 10 miles, increasing pace every 2 miles

Pacing Information: Start at a comfortable, easy pace for the first 2 miles. Increase your pace to a moderately hard effort for the next 2 miles, and then finish the last 2 miles at a challenging, near-maximum effort.

Cadence Commander Workout Type: Cadence
Run For 30 minutes:

- Focus on maintaining a cadence of 180 steps per minute

Pacing Information: Adjust your running speed to maintain the target cadence. This workout is designed to help improve running efficiency and form.

Rolling Rhythms Workout Type: Intervals
10 rounds:

- Run 400 meters

- Rest 1:1 (rest the same amount of time it took to complete the previous 400 meters)

*Pacing Information: Aim to run each interval at a fast pace, around 85-90% of your maximum effort. Use the rest periods to recover and focus on maintaining a consistent

pace for each interval.*

Recovery Ramble Workout Type: Recovery Run
For time:

- Run 3 miles

Pacing Information: Run at a comfortable, easy pace, about 50-60% of your maximum effort. This run is meant to be relaxing and rejuvenating.

Intense Intervals Workout Type: Intervals 5 rounds:

- Run 1 mile

- Rest 5 minutes

Pacing Information: Aim to run each mile at a fast, challenging pace. Use the 5-minute rest periods to recover.

Tempo Tamer Workout Type: Tempo Run
For time:

- Run 6 miles

Pacing Information: Run at a comfortably hard pace, about 75-80% of your maximum effort. Try to maintain a consistent pace throughout the entire run.

Speedy Sprints Workout Type: Intervals
10 rounds:

- Sprint 50 meters

- Walk 50 meters

Pacing Information: Run each sprint at near-maximum effort. Use the walk back as your recovery period.

Long Haul Workout Type: Long Slow Distance

For time:

- Run 20 miles

Pacing Information: Run at a comfortable, conversational pace, about 60-70% of your maximum effort. Focus on maintaining a steady rhythm and staying relaxed throughout the run.

The Two Miler Workout Type: Time Trial

For time:

- Run 2 miles

Pacing Information: Aim to complete the 2 miles as fast as possible, pushing yourself to maintain a high intensity throughout the run. This is a test of your speed and endurance.

Fast and Furious Fartlek Workout Type: Fartlek

For 40 minutes:

- Alternate between 3 minutes of easy running and 2 minutes of fast running

Pacing Information: During the easy running segments, maintain a relaxed and comfortable pace. During the fast segments, aim for 85-90% of your maximum effort.

AMRAP Workouts

AMRAP stands for "As Many Rounds (or Reps) As Possible". These workouts are a staple of CrossFit and Cross Training methodologies and they're designed to push your metabolic conditioning to its limits. AMRAP workouts are timed, usually lasting 10, 15, or 20 minutes, though they can be shorter or longer. The goal is to complete as many rounds or repetitions of the given exercises within the set timeframe, while maintaining good form. Because you're trying to fit in as many reps or rounds as possible, these workouts are intense and fast-paced, but also highly rewarding. They can involve any number of exercises, from bodyweight movements to barbell lifts, and the versatility of AMRAPs means they can be adapted to suit any fitness level. Let's get started with a few sample workouts to illustrate this concept.

Metal Mover 12 minutes:

- 8 Power Cleans (135/96 lbs - 61/43 kg)

- 16 Box Jumps (24/20")

Triplet Terror 15 minutes:

- 10 Wall Balls (20/14 lbs - 9/6 kg)

- 15 Kettlebell Swings (53/35 lbs - 24/16 kg)

- 20 Double Unders

Squat Squad 20 minutes:

- 5 Front Squats (135/96 lbs - 61/43 kg)

- 10 Toes-to-Bar

- 15 Calorie Row

Lifting Ladder 10 minutes:

- 2 Thrusters (95/65 lbs - 43/30 kg)

- 2 Pull-ups

- 4 Thrusters (95/65 lbs - 43/30 kg)

- 4 Pull-ups
  Continue adding 2 reps to each exercise per round.

Barbell Burner 18 minutes:

- 7 Deadlifts (185/132 lbs - 84/60 kg)

- 14 Push-ups

- 21 Double Unders

Cardio Craze 16 minutes:

- 10 Calorie BikeErg

- 15 Dumbbell Snatches (50/35 lbs - 23/16 kg)

Pull and Push 15 minutes:

- 5 Pull-ups

- 10 Push-ups

- 15 Air Squats

Burpee Bonanza 12 minutes:

- 10 Burpees

- 20 Double Unders

Core Crusher 15 minutes:

- 20 Sit-ups

- 10 Toes-to-Bar

- 5 Handstand Push-ups

Jump and Jerk 20 minutes:

- 10 Box Jumps (24/20")

- 5 Clean and Jerks (135/96 lbs - 61/43 kg)

Thruster Thunder 14 minutes:

- 7 Thrusters (95/65 lbs - 43/30 kg)

- 7 Pull-ups

Jump and Jerk 15 minutes:

- 15 Double Unders

- 10 Push Jerks (135/96 lbs - 61/43 kg)

Rowing Rumble 20 minutes:

- 500m Row

- 5 Devil Press (2x 50/35 lbs - 23/16 kg)

- 20 Wall Balls (20/14 lbs - 9/6 kg)

Snatch and Swing 18 minutes:

- 10 Power Snatches (95/65 lbs - 43/30 kg)

- 15 Kettlebell Swings (53/35 lbs - 24/16 kg)

HSPU Hustle 12 minutes:

- 5 Handstand Push-ups

- 10 Dumbbell Snatches (53/35 lbs - 24/16 kg)

Bike and Burpee 10 minutes:

- 10 Calorie BikeErg

- 10 Burpees

Climb and Clean 17 minutes:

- 1 Rope Climb

- 5 Power Cleans (135/96 lbs - 61/43 kg)

Double Under Delight 16 minutes:

- 30 Double Unders

- 15 Deadlifts (185/132 lbs - 84/60 kg)

Pull-up Power 20 minutes:

- 5 Pull-ups

- 10 Push-ups

- 15 Squats

Squat and Swing 15 minutes:

- 10 Goblet Squats (53/35 lbs - 24/16 kg)

- 15 Kettlebell Swings (53/35 lbs - 24/16 kg)

Row and Rope 18 minutes:

- 250m Row

- 1 Rope Climb

Dumbbell Dash 12 minutes:

- 10 Dumbbell Snatches (53/35 lbs - 24/16 kg)

- 10 Box Jumps (24/20")

Bench and Bike 16 minutes:

- 8 Bench Presses (135/96 lbs - 61/43 kg)

- 12 Calorie BikeErg

Wall Ball Wonder 20 minutes:

- 20 Wall Balls (20/14 lbs - 9/6 kg)

- 20 Double Unders

Snatch and Squat 14 minutes:

- 10 Power Snatches (95/65 lbs - 43/30 kg)

- 10 Overhead Squats (95/65 lbs - 43/30 kg)

Calorie Crush 15 minutes:

- 15 Calorie Row

- 10 Toes-to-bars

- 5 Burpees-to-bar

Dip and Drive 13 minutes:

- 10 Ring Dips

- 10 Kettlebell Swings (53/35 lbs - 24/16 kg)

Elevated Effort 20 minutes:

- 5 Handstand Push-ups

- 10 Lunges

- 15 Air Squats

- 20 Sit-ups

Clean and Climb 16 minutes:

- 5 Power Cleans (135/96 lbs - 61/43 kg)

- 1 Rope Climb

Thruster Trio 15 minutes:

- 7 Thrusters (95/65 lbs - 43/30 kg)

- 7 Box Jumps (24/20")

- 7 Kettlebell Swings (53/35 lbs - 24/16 kg)

Quad Quake 18 minutes:

- 10 Double Unders

- 10 Push Jerks (135/96 lbs - 61/43 kg)

- 10 Toes-to-bars

- 10 Dumbbell Snatches (53/35 lbs - 24/16 kg)

Rowing Rampage 20 minutes:

- 500m Row

- 15 Wall Balls (20/14 lbs - 9/6 kg)

- 10 Pull-ups

Squat Snatch Swing 16 minutes:

- 5 Overhead Squats (95/65 lbs - 43/30 kg)

- 10 Power Snatches (95/65 lbs - 43/30 kg)

- 15 Kettlebell Swings (53/35 lbs - 24/16 kg)

Climb Clean and Carry 14 minutes:

- 1 Rope Climb

- 5 Power Cleans (135/96 lbs - 61/43 kg)

- 100m Farmer's Walk (2x 50/35 lbs - 23/16 kg)

Jump Rope and Jerk 15 minutes:

- 30 Double Unders

- 15 Push Jerks (135/96 lbs - 61/43 kg)

- 15 Calorie Row

Push Pull and Pedal 12 minutes:

- 10 Push-ups

- 10 Pull-ups

- 10 Calorie BikeErg

Swing Squat and Step 20 minutes:

- 10 Kettlebell Swings (53/35 lbs - 24/16 kg)

- 10 Goblet Squats(53/35 lbs - 24/16 kg)

- 10 Box Step-ups (24/20")

Row Rope and Run 18 minutes:

- 250m Row

- 1 Rope Climb

- 200m Run

Dumbbell Drive 14 minutes:

- 10 Dumbbell Snatches (50/35 lbs - 23/16 kg)

- 10 Dumbbell Goblet Squats (50/35 lbs - 23/16 kg)

- 10 Dumbbell Push Presses (50/35 lbs - 23/16 kg)

Bench Bike and Burpee 16 minutes:

- 8 Bench Presses (135/96 lbs - 61/43 kg)

- 12 Calorie BikeErg

- 8 Burpees

Wall Ball Wonder 20 minutes:

- 20 Wall Balls (20/14 lbs - 9/6 kg)

- 20 Double Unders

- 10 Toes-to-bars

Snatch Squat and Swing 14 minutes:

- 5 Power Snatches (95/65 lbs - 43/30 kg)

- 5 Overhead Squats (95/65 lbs - 43/30 kg)

- 15 Kettlebell Swings (53/35 lbs - 24/16 kg)

Row Raise and Run 15 minutes:

- 15 Calorie Row

- 10 Toes-to-bars

- 200m Run

Dip Drive and Double 13 minutes:

- 10 Ring Dips

- 10 Kettlebell Swings (53/35 lbs - 24/16 kg)

- 30 Double Unders

Elevated Effort 20 minutes:

- 5 Handstand Push-ups

- 15 Air Squats

- 10 Pull-ups

Clean Climb and Carry 16 minutes:

- 5 Power Cleans (135/96 lbs - 61/43 kg)

- 1 Rope Climb

- 100m Farmer's Walk (2x 50/35 lbs - 23/16 kg)

Bike Burpee and Box 12 minutes:

- 10 Calorie BikeErg

- 10 Burpees

- 10 Box Jumps (24/20")

Deadlift and Double 15 minutes:

- 10 Deadlifts (225/155 lbs - 102/70 kg)

- 30 Double Unders

- 10 Pull-ups

Push Press and Pedal 14 minutes:

- 10 Push Presses (135/96 lbs - 61/43 kg)

- 10 Calorie BikeErg

- 10 Toes-to-bars

EMOM Workouts

EMOM is a popular acronym in the world of CrossFit and Cross Training that stands for "Every Minute On the Minute." In these workouts, you start a new round of exercises at the beginning of every minute, and whatever time you have left in that minute after completing the round is your rest period. If a round takes you 40 seconds, you get 20 seconds of rest. If a round takes 50 seconds, you only get 10 seconds of rest.

This format can lead to intense, challenging workouts that test your speed, endurance, and ability to recover quickly. EMOM workouts are great for skill development, conditioning, and can be easily scaled to any fitness level. They are also fantastic for keeping workouts within a specific time frame.

E2MOM and E3MOM are variations of EMOM workouts. E2MOM stands for "Every 2 Minutes On the Minute" and E3MOM stands for "Every 3 Minutes On the Minute". These types of workouts provide a longer time frame to perform more complex or heavier sets of exercises, and also provide more rest time between sets.

Let's dive into the world of EMOM workouts:

Squat Snatch Serenity EMOM for 10 minutes:

- 2 Squat Snatches (135/96 lbs - 61/43 kg)

Thruster Thrill E2MOM for 20 minutes:

- 5 Thrusters (95/65 lbs - 43/30 kg)

Pull-up Power EMOM for 12 minutes:

- 5 Pull-ups

Deadlift Delight E3MOM for 15 minutes:

- 3 Deadlifts (225/155 lbs - 102/70 kg)

Kettlebell Kick EMOM for 14 minutes:

- 10 Kettlebell Swings (53/35 lbs - 24/16 kg)

Olympic Encore E2MOM for 20 minutes:

- 3 Power Cleans (155/110 lbs - 70/50 kg)

- 3 Hang Squat Cleans (155/110 lbs - 70/50 kg)

- 3 Push Jerks (155/110 lbs - 70/50 kg)

Burpee Burn EMOM for 15 minutes:

- 15 Burpees

Double Trouble E3MOM for 21 minutes:

- 75 Double Unders

- 15 Toes-to-bar

Muscle Up Magic EMOM for 20 minutes:

- 5 Muscle Ups

Rowing Rumble E2MOM for 20 minutes:

- Row 500 meters

Handstand Hustle EMOM for 15 minutes:

- 45 seconds Handstand Hold

Jumping Jack Flash EMOM for 20 minutes:

- 50 Jumping Jacks

Wall Ball Wonder E3MOM for 18 minutes:

- 30 Wall Balls (20/14 lbs - 9/6 kg)

Box Jump Bonanza EMOM for 16 minutes:

- 15 Box Jumps (24/20")

Goblet Goodness E2MOM for 16 minutes:

- 10 Goblet Squats (50/35 lbs - 23/16 kg)

- 10 Kettlebell Swings (50/35 lbs - 23/16 kg)

Kettlebell Cascade EMOM for 20 minutes:

- 12 Kettlebell Swings (53/35 lbs - 24/16 kg)

- 10 Goblet Squats (53/35 lbs - 24/16 kg)

- 15 Kettlebell Deadlifts (53/35 lbs - 24/16 kg)

- Rest

Jumping Jacks Jamboree EMOM for 36 minutes:

- 20 Jumping Jacks

- 15 Air Squats

- 10 Push Ups

- 5 Burpees

Jump and Jive E3MOM for 33 minutes:

- 20 Double Unders

- 15 Wall Walks

- 10 Box Jumps (24/20")

Kettlebell Cruise EMOM for 45 minutes:

- 12 Kettlebell Swings (53/35 lbs - 24/16 kg)

- 10 Goblet Squats (53/35 lbs - 24/16 kg)

- 15 Kettlebell Deadlifts (53/35 lbs - 24/16 kg)

- 20 Double Unders

Dumbbell Dash EMOM for 40 minutes:

- 10 Dumbbell Snatches (50/35 lbs - 23/16 kg)

- 12 Dumbbell Thrusters (50/35 lbs - 23/16 kg)

- 14 Dumbbell Lunges (50/35 lbs - 23/16 kg)

Rowing Rhythm E2MOM for 36 minutes:

- 15 Calorie Row

- 10 Thrusters (95/65 lbs - 43/30 kg)

- 5 Pull-ups

Barbell Blast E3MOM for 21 minutes:

- 5 Power Cleans (135/96 lbs - 61/43 kg)

- 10 Front Squats (135/96 lbs - 61/43 kg)

- 15 Push Press (135/96 lbs - 61/43 kg)

Sweat Storm E3MOM for 33 minutes:

- 20 Calorie BikeErg

- 15 Toes-to-bar

- 10 Overhead Squats (95/65 lbs - 43/30 kg)

Devil's Dance E2MOM for 40 minutes:

- 5 Dumbbell Devil Presses (2x 50/35 lbs - 23/16 kg)

- 10 Dumbbell Lunges (2x 50/35 lbs - 23/16 kg)

- 20 Double Unders

Pull and Push EMOM for 30 minutes:

- 10 Pull-ups

- 12 Push-ups

- 14 Air Squats

- Rest

Row and Throw E3MOM for 33 minutes:

- 12 Calorie Row

- 10 Wall Balls (20/14 lbs - 9/6 kg)

- 8 Dumbbell Devil Presses (2x 50/35 lbs - 23/16 kg)

Dumbbell Dazzle EMOM for 27 minutes:

- 10 Dumbbell Deadlifts (2x 50/35 lbs - 23/16 kg)

- 10 Dumbbell Hang Cleans (2x 50/35 lbs - 23/16 kg)

- 10 Dumbbell Shoulder-to-Overhead (2x 50/35 lbs - 23/16 kg)

Box Jump Bash E2MOM for 20 minutes:

- 10 Box Jumps (24/20")

- 12 Dumbbell Snatches (2x 50/35 lbs - 23/16 kg)

Swing and Squat EMOM for 45 minutes:

- 20 Kettlebell Swings (53/35 lbs - 24/16 kg)

- 20 Goblet Squats (53/35 lbs - 24/16 kg)

- 20 Kettlebell Deadlifts (2x 53/35 lbs - 24/16 kg)

- Rest

Overhead Odyssey E3MOM for 36 minutes:

- 5 Power Snatches (135/96 lbs - 61/43 kg)

- 10 Overhead Squats (135/96 lbs - 61/43 kg)

- 15 Push Presses (135/96 lbs - 61/43 kg)

Cycling Circuit EMOM for 30 minutes:

- 20 Calorie BikeErg

- 15 Toes-to-bar

- 10 Dumbbell Devil Presses (2x 50/35 lbs - 23/16 kg)

Jump Rope Joy E2MOM for 30 minutes:

- 30 Double Unders

- 10 Dumbbell Thrusters (2x 50/35 lbs - 23/16 kg)

- 30 Double Unders

Barbell Bonanza E3MOM for 33 minutes:

- 5 Clean and Jerks (135/96 lbs - 61/43 kg)

- 10 Front Squats (135/96 lbs - 61/43 kg)

- 15 Deadlifts (135/96 lbs - 61/43 kg)

LADDER WORKOUTS

In the realm of Cross Training and CrossFit, Ladder Workouts present a unique challenge. These workouts operate on an ascending or descending rep scheme, testing your physical and mental endurance as you either "climb up" or "go down" the ladder. The beauty of ladder workouts lies in their scalability and versatility; they can be adapted to any fitness level and incorporate any exercise, from bodyweight movements to weighted exercises.

Ladder workouts are known for their intense ability to build strength, endurance, and cardiovascular fitness. They offer a unique way to mix up your training routine, keep you engaged, and push your limits. Whether you're new to Cross Training or CrossFit or an experienced athlete, ladder workouts will surely provide a fresh perspective to your training regimen.

Now, let's dive into the ladder and challenge ourselves with these engaging workouts.

Burpee Beatdown 10-9-8-7-6-5-4-3-2-1 reps for time:

- Burpees

- Dumbbell Devil Press (2x 50/35 lbs - 23/16 kg)

Deadlift Drive 1-2-3-4-5-6-7-8-9-10 reps for time:

- Deadlifts (225/155 lbs - 102/70 kg)

- Box Jumps (24/20")

Thruster Thunder 10-9-8-7-6-5-4-3-2-1 reps for time:

- Thrusters (95/65 lbs - 43/30 kg)

- Pull-ups

Squat Serenade 1-2-3-4-5-6-7-8-9-10 reps for time:

- Back Squats (135/96 lbs - 61/43 kg)

- Toes-to-bar

Climbing the Kettlebell 10-9-8-7-6-5-4-3-2-1 reps for time:

- Kettlebell Swings (53/35 lbs - 24/16 kg)

- Goblet Squats (53/35 lbs - 24/16 kg)

Kettlebell Cascade 10-20-30-40-50-40-30-20-10 reps for time:

- Kettlebell Swings (53/35 lbs - 24/16 kg)

- Pull-ups

Row Rampage 10-20-30-20-10 reps for time:

- Calories on the Rower

- Wall Balls (20/14 lbs - 9/6 kg)

Squat Therapy 10-9-8-7-6-5-4-3-2-1 reps for time of:

- Air Squats

- Push Presses (135/96 lbs - 61/43 kg)

Row and Flow 1-2-3-4-5-6-5-4-3-2-1 reps for time of:

- Calories on the Rower

- Wall Balls (20/14 lbs - 9/6 kg)

Barbell Blitz 10-8-6-4-2 reps for time of:

- Power Cleans (135/96 lbs - 61/43 kg)

- Handstand Push-ups

Double Devil reps for time of:

- 1-2-3-4-5-4-3-2-1 Dumbbell Devil Presses (2x 50/35 lbs - 23/16 kg)

- 2-4-6-8-10-8-6-4-2 Toes-to-bars

Burpee Bonanza 3-6-9-12-15-12-9-6-3 reps for time of:

- Burpees

- Pull-ups

Thruster Thunder 10-9-8-7-6-5-4-3-2-1 reps for time of:

- Thrusters (95/65 lbs - 43/30 kg)

- Double-unders

Row and Go 2-4-6-8-10-8-6-4-2 reps for time of:

- Calories on the Rower

- Wall Balls (20/14 lbs - 9/6 kg)

Power Play 10-8-6-4-2 reps for time of:

- Power Snatches (115/81 lbs - 52/37 kg)

- Box Jumps (24/20")

Deadlift Drive 1-2-3-4-5-6-5-4-3-2-1 reps for time of:

- Deadlifts (225/155 lbs - 102/70 kg)

- Chest-to-bar Pull-ups

Squat and Swing 5-10-15-20-25-20-15-10-5 reps for time of:

- Air Squats

- Kettlebell Swings (53/35 lbs - 24/16 kg)

Press and Push 10-9-8-7-6-5-4-3-2-1 reps for time of:

- Shoulder Presses (135/96 lbs - 61/43 kg)

- Push-ups

Climb and Descend 1-2-3-4-5-4-3-2-1 reps for time of:

- Muscle-ups

- Dumbbell Devil Presses (2x 50/35 lbs - 23/16 kg)

Jump and Jerk 2-4-6-8-10-8-6-4-2 reps for time of:

- Box Jumps (24/20")

- Clean and Jerks (135/96 lbs - 61/43 kg)

Lift and Lunge 10-8-6-4-2 reps for time of:

- Deadlifts (225/155 lbs - 102/70 kg)

- Walking Lunges

CHIPPER WORKOUTS

Chipper workouts are all about endurance and mental fortitude. These multi-exercise challenges are designed to test your ability to "chip away" at a high volume of reps across a variety of movements. You will encounter everything from traditional weightlifting exercises to gymnastics movements and metabolic conditioning. The goal is to complete all the reps of one movement before moving on to the next one, aiming for the fastest time possible. Although these workouts can be long and gruelling, the sense of achievement when you finish is unparalleled. As always, prioritize form and safety over speed, and scale the movements and weights as needed. Let's get chipping!

Heroic Hustle Complete for time:

- 60 Calorie Row

- 50 Toes-to-bars

- 40 Wall Balls (20/14 lbs - 9/6 kg)

- 30 Cleans (135/96 lbs - 61/43 kg)

- 20 Muscle-ups

- 10 Handstand Push-ups

Victory Voyage Complete for time:

- 100 Double Unders

- 80 Air Squats

- 60 Calorie BikeErg

- 40 Push-ups

- 20 Deadlifts (225/155 lbs - 102/70 kg)

- 10 Rope Climbs

Brick House Chipper Complete for time:

- 100 Double Unders

- 50 Wall Balls (20/14 lb)

- 40 Calorie Row

- 30 Dumbbell Devil Presses (2x 50/35 lbs - 23/16 kg)

- 20 Overhead Squats (115/81 lbs - 52/37 kg)

- 10 Muscle Ups

- 5 Rope Climbs

Titanium Tenacity Complete for time:

- 70 Kettlebell Swings (53/35 lbs - 24/16 kg)

- 60 Sit-ups

- 50 Calorie Assault Bike

- 40 Toes-to-bars

- 30 Deadlifts (225/155 lbs - 102/70 kg)

- 20 Handstand Push-ups

- 10 Bar Muscle-ups

Tenacious Trek Complete for time:

- 75 Kettlebell Swings (53/35 lbs - 24/16 kg)

- 60 Box Jumps (24/20")

- 45 Dumbbell Snatches (50/35 lbs - 23/16 kg)

- 30 Pull-ups

- 15 Thrusters (135/96 lbs - 61/43 kg)

- 800m Run

Mettle Master Complete for time:

- 800m Run

- 60 Dumbbell Snatches (50/35 lbs - 23/16 kg)

- 50 Pull-ups

- 40 Box Jumps (24/20")

- 30 Thrusters (95/65 lbs - 43/30 kg)

- 20 Burpees Over the Bar

- 10 Clean and Jerks (135/96 lbs - 61/43 kg)

Prowess Pyramid Complete for time:

- 100 Calorie Ski Erg

- 90 Double Unders

- 80 Wall Balls (20/14 lbs - 9/6 kg)

- 70 Kettlebell Swings (53/35 lbs - 24/16 kg)

- 60 Sit-ups

- 50 Calorie Row

- 40 Toes-to-bars

- 30 Overhead Squats (95/65 lbs - 43/30 kg)

- 20 Handstand Push-ups

- 10 Muscle Ups

- 5 Deadlifts (225/155 lbs - 102/70 kg)

Resilience Rumble Complete for time:

- 2000m Row

- 100 Double Unders

- 80 Calorie BikeErg

- 60 Dumbbell Thrusters (2x 50/35 lbs - 23/16 kg)

- 40 Chest-to-bar Pull-ups

- 20 Strict Handstand Push-ups

- 10 Snatches (135/96 lbs - 61/43 kg)

- 5 Ring Muscle-ups

Endurance Engine Complete for time:

- 1 Mile Run

- 100 Push-ups

- 90 Kettlebell Swings (135/96 lbs - 61/43 kg)

- 800 Meter Row

- 70 Wall Balls (20/14 lbs - 9/6 kg)

- 60 Calorie BikeErg

- 50 Box Jumps (24/20")

- 40 Toes-to-bars

- 30 Clean and Jerks (135/96 lbs - 61/43 kg)

- 20 Handstand Push-ups

- 10 Bar Muscle-ups

Toughness Titan Complete for time:

- 100 Double Unders

- 90 Calorie Ski Erg

- 80 Air Squats

- 70 Sit-ups

- 60 Calorie Row

- 50 Dumbbell Snatches (50/35 lbs - 23/16 kg)

- 40 Pull-ups

- 30 Thrusters (95/65 lbs - 43/30 kg)

- 20 Burpees Over the Bar

- 10 Clean and Jerks (135/96 lbs - 61/43 kg)

- 1 Mile Run

Gallant Gallop Complete for time:

- 50 Calorie Ski Erg

- 40 Toes-to-bars

- 30 Overhead Squats (115/81 lbs - 52/37 kg)

- 20 Handstand Push-ups

- 10 Bar Muscle-ups

- 1 Mile Run

Fortitude Force Complete for time:

- 2000m Row

- 90 Double Unders

- 80 Wall Balls (20/14 lbs - 9/6 kg)

- 70 Kettlebell Swings (135/96 lbs - 61/43 kg)

- 60 Sit-ups

- 50 Calorie BikeErg

- 40 Toes-to-bars

- 30 Overhead Squats (95/65 lbs - 43/30 kg)

- 20 Handstand Push-ups

- 10 Muscle Ups

Perseverance Powerhouse Complete for time:

- 1 Mile Run

- 100 Dumbbell Snatches (50/35 lbs - 23/16 kg)

- 90 Push-ups

- 800 Meter Row

- 70 Wall Balls (20/14 lbs - 9/6 kg)

- 60 Calorie BikeErg

- 50 Box Jumps (24/20")

- 40 Pull-ups

- 30 Thrusters (95/65 lbs - 43/30 kg)

- 20 Burpees Over the Bar

- 10 Bar Muscle-ups

Relentless Rally Complete for time:

- 100 Calorie Ski Erg

- 90 Double Unders

- 80 Wall Balls (20/14 lbs - 9/6 kg)

- 70 Kettlebell Swings (135/96 lbs - 61/43 kg)

- 60 Sit-ups

- 50 Calorie Row

- 40 Toes-to-bars

- 30 Overhead Squats (95/65 lbs - 43/30 kg)

- 20 Handstand Push-ups

- 10 Muscle Ups

- 1 Mile Run

Strength Surge Complete for time:

- 2000m Row

- 90 Double Unders

- 80 Air Squats

- 70 Sit-ups

- 60 Calorie BikeErg

- 50 Dumbbell Snatches (50/35 lbs - 23/16 kg)

- 40 Pull-ups

- 30 Thrusters (95/65 lbs - 43/30 kg)

- 20 Burpees Over the Bar

- 10 Clean and Jerks (135/96 lbs - 61/43 kg)

Mighty Marathon Complete for time:

- 60 Calorie Row

- 60 Burpees Over the Bar

- 60 Double Unders

- 60 Power Cleans (135/96 lbs - 61/43 kg)

- 60 Pull-ups

- 60 Overhead Squats (135/96 lbs - 61/43 kg)

Vigor Vortex Complete for time:

- 1 Mile Run

- 100 Push-ups

- 90 Kettlebell Swings (135/96 lbs - 61/43 kg)

- 800 Meter Row

- 70 Wall Balls (20/14 lbs - 9/6 kg)

- 60 Calorie BikeErg

- 50 Box Jumps (24/20")

- 40 Toes-to-bars

- 30 Clean and Jerks (135/96 lbs - 61/43 kg)

- 20 Handstand Push-ups

- 10 Bar Muscle-ups

Determination Dynamo Complete for time:

- 100 Double Unders

- 90 Calorie Ski Erg

- 80 Air Squats

- 70 Sit-ups

- 60 Calorie Row

- 50 Dumbbell Snatches (50/35 lbs - 23/16 kg)

- 40 Pull-ups

- 30 Thrusters (95/65 lbs - 43/30 kg)

- 20 Burpees Over the Bar

- 10 Clean and Jerks (135/96 lbs - 61/43 kg)

- 1 Mile Run

Valor Vanguard Complete for time:

- 2000m Row

- 90 Double Unders

- 80 Wall Balls (20/14 lbs - 9/6 kg)

- 70 Kettlebell Swings (135/96 lbs - 61/43 kg)

- 60 Sit-ups

- 50 Calorie BikeErg

- 40 Toes-to-bars

- 30 Overhead Squats (95/65 lbs - 43/30 kg)

- 20 Handstand Push-ups

- 10 Muscle Ups

Grit Grinder Complete for time:

- 1 Mile Run

- 100 Dumbbell Snatches (50/35 lbs - 23/16 kg)

- 90 Push-ups

- 800 Meter Row

- 70 Wall Balls (20/14 lbs - 9/6 kg)

- 60 Calorie BikeErg

- 50 Box Jumps (24/20")

- 40 Pull-ups

- 30 Thrusters (95/65 lbs - 43/30 kg)

- 20 Burpees Over the Bar

- 10 Bar Muscle-ups

Courageous Comeback Complete for time:

- 100 Calorie Ski Erg

- 90 Double Unders

- 80 Wall Balls (95/65 lbs - 43/30 kg)

- 70 Kettlebell Snatches (135/96 lbs - 61/43 kg)

- 60 Sit-ups

- 50 Calorie Row

- 40 Toes-to-bars

- 30 Overhead Squats (95/65 lbs - 43/30 kg)

- 20 Handstand Push-ups

- 10 Muscle Ups

- 1 Mile Run

Fortitude Fury Complete for time:

- 100 Calorie Row

- 100 Double Unders

- 100 Wall Balls (95/65 lbs - 43/30 kg)

- 100 Kettlebell Swings (135/96 lbs - 61/43 kg)

- 100 Sit-ups

Bravery Blaze Complete for time:

- 2000m Row

- 90 Double Unders

- 80 Air Squats

- 70 Sit-ups

- 60 Calorie BikeErg

- 50 Dumbbell Snatches (50/35 lbs - 23/16 kg)

- 40 Pull-ups

- 30 Thrusters (95/65 lbs - 43/30 kg)

- 20 Burpees Over the Bar

- 10 Clean and Jerks (135/96 lbs - 61/43 kg)

Heroic Hustle Complete for time:

- 1 Mile Run

- 100 Push-ups

- 90 Kettlebell Swings (53/35 lbs - 24/16 kg)

- 800 Meter Row

- 70 Wall Balls (20/14 lbs - 9/6 kg)

- 60 Calorie BikeErg

- 50 Box Jumps (24/20")

- 40 Toes-to-bars

- 30 Clean and Jerks (135/96 lbs - 61/43 kg)

- 20 Handstand Push-ups

- 10 Bar Muscle-ups

Invincible Ignite Complete for time:

- 100 Double Unders

- 90 Calorie Ski Erg

- 80 Air Squats

- 70 Sit-ups

- 60 Calorie Row

- 50 Dumbbell Squat Snatches (50/35 lbs - 23/16 kg)

- 40 Pull-ups

- 30 Dumbbell Thrusters(2x 50/35 lbs - 23/16 kg)

- 20 Burpees Over the Bar

- 10 Dumbbell Clean and Jerks (2x 50/35 lbs - 23/16 kg)

- 1 Mile Run

Endurance Eruption Complete for time:

- 100 Calorie Ski Erg

- 100 Dumbbell Snatches (50/35 lbs - 23/16 kg)

- 100 Air Squats

- 100 Pull-ups

- 100 Box Jumps (24/20")

Unyielding Unleash Complete for time:

- 2000m Row

- 90 Double Unders

- 80 Wall Balls (20/14 lbs - 9/6 kg)

- 70 Kettlebell Swings (70/53 lbs - 32/24 kg)

- 60 Weighted Sit-ups

- 50 Calorie BikeErg

- 40 Strict Toes-to-bars

- 30 Overhead Squats (135/96 lbs - 61/43 kg)

- 20 Strict Handstand Push-ups

- 10 Strict Ring Muscle Ups

Resilient Rampage Complete for time:

- 1 Mile Run

- 100 Dumbbell Snatches (50/35 lbs - 23/16 kg)

- 90 Push-ups

- 800 Meter Row

- 70 Wall Balls (20/14 lbs - 9/6 kg)

- 60 Calorie BikeErg

- 50 Box Jumps (24/20")

- 40 Pull-ups

- 30 Thrusters (95/65 lbs - 43/30 kg)

- 20 Burpees Over the Bar

- 10 Bar Muscle-ups

Gutsy Grind Complete for time:

- 100 Calorie BikeErg

- 100 Toes-to-bars

- 100 Thrusters (95/65 lbs - 43/30 kg)

- 100 Burpees Over the Bar

- 100 Double Unders

Indomitable Ignition Complete for time:

- 100 Calorie Ski Erg

- 90 Double Unders

- 80 Wall Balls (20/14 lbs - 9/6 kg)

- 70 Kettlebell Swings (53/35 lbs - 24/16 kg)

- 60 Sit-ups

- 50 Calorie Row

- 40 Toes-to-bars

- 30 Overhead Squats (95/65 lbs - 43/30 kg)

- 20 Handstand Push-ups

- 10 Muscle Ups

- 1 Mile Run

Tenacious Triumph Complete for time:

- 2000m Row

- 90 Double Unders

- 80 Air Squats

- 70 Sit-ups

- 60 Calorie BikeErg

- 50 Dumbbell Snatches (50/35 lbs - 23/16 kg)

- 40 Pull-ups

- 30 Thrusters (95/65 lbs - 43/30 kg)

- 20 Burpees Over the Bar

- 10 Clean and Jerks (135/96 lbs - 61/43 kg)

Steadfast Stampede Complete for time:

- 1 Mile Run

- 100 Push-ups

- 90 Kettlebell Swings (53/35 lbs - 24/16 kg)

- 800 Meter Row

- 70 Wall Balls (20/14 lbs - 9/6 kg)

- 60 Calorie BikeErg

- 50 Box Jumps (24/20")

- 40 Toes-to-bars

- 30 Clean and Jerks (135/96 lbs - 61/43 kg)

- 20 Handstand Push-ups

- 10 Bar Muscle-ups

Courageous Charge Complete for time:

- 100 Double Unders

- 100 Calorie Ski Erg

- 100 Air Squats

- 100 Pull-ups

- 100 Box Jumps (24/20")

Reliable Rush Complete for time:

- 100 Double Unders

- 90 Calorie Ski Erg

- 80 Air Squats

- 70 Sit-ups

- 60 Calorie Row

- 50 Dumbbell Snatches (50/35 lbs - 23/16 kg)

- 40 Pull-ups

- 30 Thrusters (95/65 lbs - 43/30 kg)

- 20 Burpees Over the Bar

- 10 Clean and Jerks (135/96 lbs - 61/43 kg)

- 1 Mile Run

TABATA WORKOUTS

Tabata workouts are an exemplary method of time-efficient, high-intensity training that can significantly boost your cardiovascular and muscular endurance. They originate from the work of Dr. Izumi Tabata, a Japanese researcher who discovered the exceptional benefits of short bursts of maximum-intensity exercise followed by brief periods of rest.

In essence, a Tabata workout consists of eight rounds of ultra-high-intensity exercises in a specific 20-seconds-on, 10-seconds-off interval. You can do a Tabata workout with almost any exercise, making it a highly versatile training method that fits effortlessly into any CrossFit or cross-training regimen. Remember, the key is to go all out during those 20-second work periods. You'll find the intensity challenging, but the results rewarding.

Now, let's introduce you to some engaging and effective Tabata workouts that will push your boundaries and elevate your fitness to new heights.

Twisted Tabata

- 8 rounds of:

  - 20 seconds of Toes-to-bars

  - 10 seconds rest

- 8 rounds of:

  - 20 seconds of Air Squats

  - 10 seconds rest

Burpee Blast

- 8 rounds of:

  - 20 seconds of Burpees

  - 10 seconds rest

- 8 rounds of:

  - 20 seconds of Push-ups

  - 10 seconds rest

Dumbbell Dynamo

- 8 rounds of:

  - 20 seconds of Dumbbell Snatches (50/35 lbs - 23/16 kg)

  - 10 seconds rest

- 8 rounds of:

- ○ 20 seconds of Dumbbell Goblet Squats (50/35 lbs - 23/16 kg)

- ○ 10 seconds rest

Kettlebell Kick

- 8 rounds of:

  - ○ 20 seconds of Kettlebell Swings (53/35 lbs - 24/16 kg)

  - ○ 10 seconds rest

- 8 rounds of:

  - ○ 20 seconds of Kettlebell Goblet Squats (53/35 lbs - 24/16 kg)

  - ○ 10 seconds rest

Row and Flow

- 8 rounds of:

  - ○ 20 seconds of Row (calories)

  - ○ 10 seconds rest

- 8 rounds of:

  - ○ 20 seconds of Wall Balls (20/14 lbs - 9/6 kg)

  - ○ 10 seconds rest

Barbell Blitz

- 8 rounds of:

  - 20 seconds of Thrusters (95/65 lbs - 43/30 kg)

  - 10 seconds rest

- 8 rounds of:

  - 20 seconds of Deadlifts (95/65 lbs - 43/30 kg)

  - 10 seconds rest

- 8 rounds of:

  - 20 seconds of Power Cleans (95/65 lbs - 43/30 kg)

  - 10 seconds rest

Jump and Slam

- 8 rounds of:

  - 20 seconds of Box Jumps (24/20")

  - 10 seconds rest

- 8 rounds of:

  - 20 seconds of Slam Balls

  - 10 seconds rest

- 8 rounds of:

  - 20 seconds of Double Unders

  - 10 seconds rest

Rope and Row

- 8 rounds of:

  - 20 seconds of Battle Rope Slams

  - 10 seconds rest

- 8 rounds of:

  - 20 seconds of Rowing (max calories)

  - 10 seconds rest

- 8 rounds of:

  - 20 seconds of Knees-to-elbows

  - 10 seconds rest

Pull and Push

- 8 rounds of:

  - 20 seconds of Pull-ups

  - 10 seconds rest

- 8 rounds of:

  - 20 seconds of Push-ups

  - 10 seconds rest

- 8 rounds of:

  - 20 seconds of Handstand Push-ups

- 10 seconds rest

Plyo Power

- 8 rounds of:

  - 20 seconds of Plyo Lunges

  - 10 seconds rest

- 8 rounds of:

  - 20 seconds of Plyo Push-ups

  - 10 seconds rest

- 8 rounds of:

  - 20 seconds of Tuck Jumps

  - 10 seconds rest

Dumbbell Devilish

- 8 rounds of:

  - 20 seconds of Dumbbell Devil Press (2x 50/35 lbs - 23/16 kg)

  - 10 seconds rest

- 8 rounds of:

  - 20 seconds of Dumbbell Front Squats (2x 50/35 lbs - 23/16 kg)

- ○ 10 seconds rest

- 8 rounds of:

  - ○ 20 seconds of Dumbbell Renegade Rows (2x 50/35 lbs - 23/16 kg)

  - ○ 10 seconds rest

Gymnastic Grinder

- 8 rounds of:

  - ○ 20 seconds of Ring Dips

  - ○ 10 seconds rest

- 8 rounds of:

  - ○ 20 seconds of Toes-to-bars

  - ○ 10 seconds rest

- 8 rounds of:

  - ○ 20 seconds of Handstand Walks

  - ○ 10 seconds rest

Kettlebell Krusher

- 8 rounds of:

  - ○ 20 seconds of Kettlebell Swings (53/35 lbs - 24/16 kg)

  - ○ 10 seconds rest

- 8 rounds of:

  - 20 seconds of Kettlebell Goblet Squats (53/35 lbs - 24/16 kg)

  - 10 seconds rest

- 8 rounds of:

  - 20 seconds of Kettlebell Snatches (53/35 lbs - 24/16 kg)

  - 10 seconds rest

Erg Assault

- 8 rounds of:

  - 20 seconds of Rowing (max distance)

  - 10 seconds rest

- 8 rounds of:

  - 20 seconds of Assault Bike (max distance)

  - 10 seconds rest

- 8 rounds of:

  - 20 seconds of SkiErg (max distance)

  - 10 seconds rest

Muscle Mayhem

- 8 rounds of:

- ○ 20 seconds of Muscle Ups

  - ○ 10 seconds rest

- 8 rounds of:

  - ○ 20 seconds of Handstand Push-ups

  - ○ 10 seconds rest

- 8 rounds of:

  - ○ 20 seconds of Pistol Squats

  - ○ 10 seconds rest

Quadruple Threat

- 8 rounds of:

  - ○ 20 seconds of Double Unders, 10 seconds rest

  - ○ 20 seconds of Air Squats, 10 seconds rest

  - ○ 20 seconds of Push-ups, 10 seconds rest

  - ○ 20 seconds of Sit-ups, 10 seconds rest

- Repeat each movement once more

Rest 1 minute and repeat twice more

Barbell Bonanza

- 8 rounds of:

  - ○ 20 seconds of Deadlifts (135/96 lbs - 61/43 kg), 10 seconds rest

- 20 seconds of Power Cleans (135/96 lbs - 61/43 kg), 10 seconds rest

- 20 seconds of Front Squats (135/96 lbs - 61/43 kg), 10 seconds rest

- 20 seconds of Push Jerks (135/96 lbs - 61/43 kg), 10 seconds rest

- Repeat each movement once more

Rest 1 minute and repeat twice more

Kettlebell Crush

- 8 rounds of:

  - 20 seconds of Kettlebell Swings (53/35 lbs - 24/16 kg), 10 seconds rest

  - 20 seconds of Kettlebell Goblet Squats (53/35 lbs - 24/16 kg), 10 seconds rest

  - 20 seconds of Kettlebell Snatches (53/35 lbs - 24/16 kg), 10 seconds rest

  - 20 seconds of Kettlebell Lunges (53/35 lbs - 24/16 kg), 10 seconds rest

- Repeat each movement once more

Rest 1 minute and repeat twice more

Gymnastic Gauntlet

- 8 rounds of:

  - 20 seconds of Handstand Push-ups, 10 seconds rest

  - 20 seconds of Pull-ups, 10 seconds rest

  - 20 seconds of Toes-to-Bar, 10 seconds rest

  - 20 seconds of Ring Dips, 10 seconds rest

- Repeat each movement once more

Rest 1 minute and repeat twice more

Dumbbell Domination

- 8 rounds of:

  - 20 seconds of Dumbbell Thrusters (50/35 lbs - 23/16 kg), 10 seconds rest

  - 20 seconds of Dumbbell Snatches (50/35 lbs - 23/16 kg), 10 seconds rest

  - 20 seconds of Dumbbell Lunges (50/35 lbs - 23/16 kg), 10 seconds rest

  - 20 seconds of Dumbbell Deadlifts (50/35 lbs - 23/16 kg), 10 seconds rest

- Repeat each movement once more

Rest 1 minute and repeat twice more

ROUNDS FOR TIME WORKOUTS

"Rounds for Time" is a popular workout format in both CrossFit and Cross Training, primarily known for its straightforward simplicity and intense demand on your endurance and strength. The goal in these workouts is to complete a specified number of rounds of a series of exercises as quickly as possible. This format pushes you to find the balance between speed and skill, requiring both efficiency in movement and the mental fortitude to push through fatigue.

The workouts in this chapter range from shorter, high-intensity blasts to longer, grinding tests of willpower. You'll encounter a diverse mix of exercises and movement combinations, designed to challenge your strength, agility, and cardiovascular fitness in unique ways. The key to success in these workouts is pacing; a strategy that allows you to maintain a high level of intensity while avoiding burnout is crucial. As always, remember to prioritize form and safety above all else.

Let's get started!

Turbulent Tides 5 rounds for time:

- 15 Box Jumps (24/20")

- 12 Dumbbell Devil Press (2x 50/35 lbs - 23/16 kg)

- 9 Toes-to-Bar

Steel Drive 3 rounds for time:

- 800m Run

- 20 Overhead Squats (95/65 lbs - 43/30 kg)

- 15 Pull-Ups

Mercury Sprint 4 rounds for time:

- 20 Double Unders

- 15 Kettlebell Swings (53/35 lbs - 24/16 kg)

- 10 Handstand Push-Ups

Blazing Comet 6 rounds for time:

- 10 Power Cleans (135/96 lbs - 61/43 kg)

- 15 Wall Balls (20/14 lbs - 9/6 kg)

Solar Flare 7 rounds for time:

- 5 Deadlifts (225/155 lbs - 102/70 kg)

- 10 Burpees Over Bar

Cosmic Race 5 rounds for time:

- 400m Run

- 15 Thrusters (95/65 lbs - 43/30 kg)

- 20 Sit-Ups

Orbit Grinder 3 rounds for time:

- 20 Dumbbell Snatches (50/35 lbs - 22.5/16 kg)

- 15 Chest-to-Bar Pull-Ups

- 400m Row

Galactic Gauntlet 4 rounds for time:

- 15 Overhead Lunges (45/25 lbs plate - 20/10 kg)

- 12 Push-Ups

- 9 Box Jumps (24/20")

Nebula Nexus 6 rounds for time:

- 10 Toes-to-Bar

- 15 Kettlebell Swings (24/16 kg - 53/35 lbs)

- 20 Double Unders

Quantum Quest 5 rounds for time:

- 15 Dumbbell Devil Press (50/35 lb - 23/16 kg)

- 12 Front Squats (135/95 lbs - 61/43 kg)

- 400m Run

Asteroid Ambush 4 rounds for time:

- 20 Wall Balls (20/14 lbs - 9/6 kg)

- 15 Box Jumps (24/20")

- 10 Power Cleans (135/95 lbs - 61/43 kg)

Lunar Launch 5 rounds for time:

- 15 Overhead Squats (95/65 lbs - 43/30 kg)

- 200m Run

- 10 Chest-to-Bar Pull-Ups

Satellite Surge 6 rounds for time:

- 5 Deadlifts (225/155 lbs - 102/70 kg)

- 10 Handstand Push-Ups

- 15 Double Unders

Solar Storm 3 rounds for time:

- 400m Row

- 20 Dumbbell Snatches (50/35 lbs - 23/16 kg)

- 10 Toes-to-Bar

Comet Clash 4 rounds for time:

- 12 Thrusters (95/65 lbs - 43/30 kg)

- 15 Box Jumps (24/20")

- 200m Run

Galaxy Grind 5 rounds for time:

- 10 Overhead Lunges (45/25 lbs plate - 20/10 kg)

- 15 Kettlebell Swings (24/16 kg - 53/35 lbs)

- 20 Sit-Ups

Orbit Overdrive 3 rounds for time:

- 400m Run

- 15 Dumbbell Devil Press (50/35 lbs – 22.5/16 kg)

- 10 Pull-Ups

Nebula Nightmare 5 rounds for time:

- 10 Front Squats (135/95 lbs - 61/43 kg)

- 15 Double Unders

- 20 Sit-Ups

Quantum Quake 4 rounds for time:

- 15 Wall Balls (20/14 lbs - 9/6 kg)

- 10 Overhead Squats (95/65 lbs - 43/30 kg)

- 200m Run

Stellar Sprint 6 rounds for time:

- 5 Power Cleans (135/95 lbs - 61/43 kg)

- 10 Box Jumps (24/20")

- 15 Double Unders

Meteor Mayhem 5 rounds for time:

- 20 Kettlebell Swings (24/16 kg – 53/35 lbs)

- 15 Toes-to-Bar

- 400m Row

Galactic Grapple 4 rounds for time:

- 10 Dumbbell Snatches (50/35 lbs - 22.5/16 kg)

- 15 Overhead Lunges (45/25 lbs plate - 20/10 kg)

- 200m Run

Pluto Plunder 6 rounds for time:

- 5 Front Squats (135/95 lbs - 61/43 kg)

- 10 Handstand Push-Ups

- 15 Box Jumps (24/20")

Cosmic Crusade 3 rounds for time:

- 400m Run

- 20 Wall Balls (20/14 lbs - 9/6 kg)

- 10 Pull-Ups

Saturn Sprint 5 rounds for time:

- 15 Overhead Squats (95/65 lbs - 43/30 kg)

- 10 Toes-to-Bar

- 200m Row

Jupiter Jump 4 rounds for time:

- 20 Double Unders

- 15 Dumbbell Devil Press (50/35 lbs - 23/16 kg)

- 10 Kettlebell Swings (24/16 kg - 53/35 lb)

Interstellar Impact 3 rounds for time:

- 800m Run

- 15 Box Jumps (24/20")

- 10 Power Cleans (135/95 lbs - 61/43 kg)

Venus Voyage 5 rounds for time:

- 10 Deadlifts (225/155 lbs - 102/70 kg)

- 15 Wall Balls (20/14 lbs - 9/6 kg)

- 20 Double Unders

Mars Mission 4 rounds for time:

- 20 Overhead Lunges (45/25 lbs plate - 20/10 kg)

- 15 Chest-to-Bar Pull-Ups

- 400m Row

Neptune Navigate 6 rounds for time:

- 5 Front Squats (135/95 lbs - 61/43 kg)

- 10 Handstand Push-Ups

- 15 Kettlebell Swings (24/16 kg - 53/35 lbs)

Supernova Surge 3 rounds for time:

- 15 Thrusters (95/65 lbs - 43/30 kg)

- 400m Run

- 10 Pull-Ups

Andromeda Adventure 5 rounds for time:

- 20 Dumbbell Snatches (50/35 lbs - 23/16 kg)

- 15 Box Jumps (24/20")

- 200m Row

Pulsar Pursuit 4 rounds for time:

- 12 Power Cleans (135/95 lbs - 61/43 kg)

- 15 Toes-to-Bar

- 20 Wall Balls (20/14 lbs - 9/6 kg)

Quasar Quest 6 rounds for time:

- 10 Deadlifts (225/155 lbs - 102/70 kg)

- 15 Double Unders

- 20 Sit-Ups

Celestial Charge 5 rounds for time:

- 400m Run

- 15 Overhead Squats (95/65 lbs - 43/30 kg)

- 10 Chest-to-Bar Pull-Ups

Orion Odyssey 4 rounds for time:

- 20 Kettlebell Swings (24/16 kg - 53/35 lb)

- 15 Dumbbell Devil Press (50/35 lbs - 23/16 kg)

- 200m Run

Vortex Venture 5 rounds for time:

- 20 Double Unders

- 15 Wall Balls (20/14 lbs - 9/6 kg)

- 10 Overhead Squats (95/65 lbs or 43/30 kg)

Nova Nomad 4 rounds for time:

- 400m Run

- 15 Dumbbell Snatches (50/35 lbs - 23/16 kg)

- 10 Toes-to-Bar

Eclipse Endeavor 3 rounds for time:

- 20 Kettlebell Swings (24/16 kg - 53/35 lb)

- 15 Box Jumps (24/20")

- 10 Power Cleans (135/95 lbs – 61/43 kg)

Pulsar Pursuit 5 rounds for time:

- 15 Deadlifts (225/155 lbs - 102/70 kg)

- 10 Handstand Push-Ups

- 400m Row

Starlight Sprint 6 rounds for time:

- 20 Wall Balls (20/14 lb - 9/6 kg)

- 15 Overhead Lunges (45/25 lbs plate - 20/10 kg)

- 10 Chest-to-Bar Pull-Ups

Astral Adventure 5 rounds for time:

- 400m Run

- 15 Dumbbell Devil Press (50/35 lbs - 23/16 kg)

- 10 Toes-to-Bar

Orion Odyssey 3 rounds for time:

- 20 Kettlebell Swings (24/16 kg - 53/35 lb)

- 15 Double Unders

- 10 Power Cleans (135/95 lb - 61/43 kg)

Stellar Soar 4 rounds for time:

- 15 Deadlifts (225/155 lbs - 102/70 kg)

- 10 Handstand Push-Ups

- 400m Row

Supernova Sprint 5 rounds for time:

- 20 Wall Balls (20/14 lb - 9/6 kg)

- 15 Overhead Lunges (45/25 lbs plate – 20/10 kg)

- 10 Chest-to-Bar Pull-Ups

Cosmic Charge 3 rounds for time:

- 400m Run

- 20 Dumbbell Snatches (50/35 lbs - 22.5/16 kg)

- 15 Toes-to-Bar

Galactic Grind 5 rounds for time:

- 15 Kettlebell Swings (24/16 kg - 53/35 lb)

- 10 Power Cleans (135/95 lbs - 61/43 kg)

- 400m Row

Meteor Mayhem 6 rounds for time:

- 20 Wall Balls (20/14 lbs - 9/6 kg)

- 15 Double Unders

- 10 Overhead Squats (95/65 lbs - 43/29.5 kg)

Solar Surge 4 rounds for time:

- 400m Run

- 15 Dumbbell Devil Press (50/35 lbs - 23/16 kg)

- 10 Chest-to-Bar Pull-Ups

Nebula Nightmare 3 rounds for time:

- 20 Kettlebell Swings (24/16 kg - 53/35 lb)

- 15 Double Unders

- 10 Power Cleans (135/95 lbs - 61/43 kg)

Couplet & Triplet Workouts

Couplet and Triplet workouts are a cornerstone of CrossFit methodology. They are designed to test your fitness and versatility by combining different movements in a single session. These workouts are so named because they involve two (Couplet) or three (Triplet) different exercises that you cycle through for a set number of rounds or time.

Couplets and Triplets are renowned for their simplicity and effectiveness. They allow for a wide range of movement patterns and energy systems to be targeted in a single workout. When programming these workouts, balance between different domains such as weightlifting, gymnastics, and monostructural (cardio) is often sought.

These workouts are superb for improving your overall conditioning and are great for those days when you're short on time but still want a challenging and comprehensive workout. Whether you are a seasoned CrossFit athlete or a beginner, couplet and triplet workouts can be scaled to suit your current level of fitness and ability. Enjoy the burn and the broad fitness gains these workouts offer!

Deadlift Dynamo 3 rounds for time:

- 10 Deadlifts (225/155 lbs - 100/70 kg)

- 20 Toes-to-bars

Squat Snatch Symphony AMRAP in 12 minutes:

- 5 Squat Snatches (135/95 lbs - 60/45 kg)

- 15 Pull-ups

Double Under Duty 4 rounds for time:

- 50 Double Unders

- 15 Overhead Squats (95/65 lbs - 45/30 kg)

Barbell Burpee Blast For time:

- 21-15-9

- Burpees over Bar

- Thrusters (95/65 lbs - 45/30 kg)

Kettlebell Khaos AMRAP in 15 minutes:

- 20 Kettlebell Swings (53/35 lbs - 24/16 kg)

- 200 meter Run

Wall Ball Wonder 3 rounds for time:

- 30 Wall Balls (20/14 lbs - 9/6 kg)

- 15 Power Cleans (135/95 lbs - 60/45 kg)

Rowing Rampage AMRAP in 20 minutes:

- 500 meter Row

- 15 Dumbbell Devil Presses (50/35 lbs - 22.5/16 kg)

Jumping Jack Flash For time:

- 100 Double Unders

- 50 Sit-ups

- 25 Push Press (115/80 lbs - 50/35 kg)

Box Jump Bonanza 5 rounds for time:

- 15 Box Jumps (24/20 inch)

- 10 Overhead Squats (115/80 lbs - 50/35 kg)

Dumbbell Devil Dance AMRAP in 10 minutes:

- 10 Dumbbell Devil Presses (50/35 lbs - 22.5/16 kg)

- 20 Alternating Dumbbell Lunges

Pull-up Power 3 rounds for time:

- 15 Pull-ups

- 30 Air Squats

Toes-to-Bar Tango AMRAP in 8 minutes:

- 10 Toes-to-bars

- 20 Kettlebell Swings (53/35 lbs - 24/16 kg)

Clean and Jerk Jive For time:

- 10-9-8-7-6-5-4-3-2-1

- Clean and Jerks (135/95 lbs - 60/45 kg)

- 50 Double Unders after each set

Front Squat Frenzy 5 rounds for time:

- 10 Front Squats (135/95 lbs - 60/45 kg)

- 200 meter Run

Burpee Box Jump Beatdown AMRAP in 14 minutes:

- 10 Burpee Box Jumps (24/20")

- 15 Wall Balls (20/14 lbs - 9/6 kg)

Thruster Thunder For time:

- 21-15-9

- Thrusters (95/65 lbs - 45/30 kg)

- Pull-ups

Muscle-up Madness AMRAP in 16 minutes:

- 5 Muscle-ups

- 10 Handstand Push-ups

- 15 Kettlebell Swings (53/35 lbs - 24/16 kg)

Sit-up Slam 3 rounds for time:

- 50 Sit-ups

- 25 Overhead Squats (95/65 lbs - 45/30 kg)

Double Under Delight AMRAP in 10 minutes:

- 100 Double Unders

- 20 Alternating Dumbbell Snatches (50/35 lbs - 23/16 kg)

Push Press Party 5 rounds for time:

- 15 Push Press (115/80 lbs - 50/35 kg)

- 30 Air Squats

Rowing Rumble For time:

- 1000 meter Row

- 50 Thrusters (95/65 lbs - 45/30 kg)

- 30 Pull-ups

Squat Clean Sequence AMRAP in 12 minutes:

- 10 Squat Cleans (135/95 lbs - 60/45 kg)

- 20 Toes-to-bars

Kettlebell Krush 3 rounds for time:

- 20 Kettlebell Snatches (53/35 lbs - 24/16 kg)

- 400 meter Run

Wall Ball Whirl AMRAP in 15 minutes:

- 30 Wall Balls (20/14 lbs - 9/6 kg)

- 15 Toes-to-bars

Jumping Jive For time:

- 150 Double Unders

- 75 Sit-ups

- 50 Push Press (115/80 lbs - 50/35 kg)

Box Jump Blitz 5 rounds for time:

- 20 Box Jumps (24/20")

- 10 Overhead Lunges (45/25 lbs - 20/10 kg Plate)

Dumbbell Devil Dash AMRAP in 9 minutes:

- 15 Dumbbell Devil Presses (50/35 lbs - 22.5/16 kg)

- 30 Double Unders

Pull-up Pounce 3 rounds for time:

- 20 Pull-ups

- 40 Air Squats

Toes-to-Bar Twist AMRAP in 7 minutes:

- 15 Toes-to-bars

- 30 Kettlebell Goblet Squats (53/35 lbs - 24/16 kg)

Clean and Jerk Carnival For time:

- 1-2-3-4-5-6-7-8-9-10

- Clean and Jerks (135/95 lbs - 60/45 kg)

- 50 Double Unders after each set

Front Squat Fiesta 5 rounds for time:

- 15 Front Squats (135/95 lbs - 60/45 kg)

- 300 meter Run

Burpee Box Jump Bash AMRAP in 13 minutes:

- 15 Burpee Box Jumps (24/20")

- 20 Wall Balls (20/14 lbs - 9/6 kg)

Thruster Tempest For time:

- 18-15-12

- Thrusters (95/65 lbs - 45/30 kg)

- Chest-to-bar Pull-ups

Muscle-up Mania AMRAP in 15 minutes:

- 7 Muscle-ups

- 14 Handstand Push-ups

- 21 Kettlebell Swings (53/35 lbs - 24/16 kg)

Sit-up Sizzle 3 rounds for time:

- 60 Sit-ups

- 30 Overhead Lunges (45/25 lbs - 20/10 kg Plate)

Double Under Dazzle AMRAP in 11 minutes:

- 150 Double Unders

- 30 Alternating Dumbbell Snatches (50/35 lbs - 22.5/16 kg)

Push Press Parade 5 rounds for time:

- 20 Push Press (115/80 lbs - 50/35 kg)

- 40 Double Unders

Rowing Riot For time:

- 2000 meter Row

- 50 Thrusters (95/65 lbs - 45/30 kg)

- 30 Chest-to-bar Pull-ups

Squat Clean Spectacle AMRAP in 14 minutes:

- 15 Squat Cleans (135/95 lbs - 60/45 kg)

- 30 Toes-to-bars

Kettlebell Kick 3 rounds for time:

- 25 Kettlebell Snatches (53/35 lbs - 24/16 kg)

- 500 meter Run

Wall Ball Waltz AMRAP in 18 minutes:

- 40 Wall Balls (20/14 lbs - 9/6 kg)

- 20 Toes-to-bars

Deadlift Delight 4 rounds for time:

- 10 Deadlifts (225/155 lbs - 100/70 kg)

- 20 Handstand Push-ups

Power Snatch Party AMRAP in 10 minutes:

- 5 Power Snatches (135/95 lbs - 60/45 kg)

- 10 Burpees Over the Bar

Row and Swing 5 rounds for time:

- 500 meter Row

- 25 Kettlebell Swings (53/35 lbs - 24/16 kg)

Lunge and Lift For time:

- 100 Overhead Walking Lunges (45/25 lbs - 20/10 kg Plate)

- 50 Chest-to-bar Pull-ups

- 100 Double Unders

Barbell Burpee Bonanza AMRAP in 15 minutes:

- 10 Bar-facing Burpees

- 15 Power Cleans (135/95 lbs - 60/45 kg)

- 20 Box Jumps (24/20")

Jump Rope Joyride For time:

- 200 Double Unders

- 100 Air Squats

- 50 Push Press (115/80 lbs - 50/35 kg)

Tire Flip Frenzy 3 rounds for time:

- 20 Tire Flips

- 400 meter Run

Muscle-up Madness AMRAP in 12 minutes:

- 5 Muscle-ups

- 10 Handstand Push-ups

- 15 Kettlebell Swings (70/53 lbs - 32/24 kg)

Sit-up Sprint 4 rounds for time:

- 50 Sit-ups

- 25 Overhead Lunges (45/25 lbs - 20/10 kg Plate)

Double Under Dash AMRAP in 8 minutes:

- 100 Double Unders

- 20 Alternating Dumbbell Snatches (50/35 lbs - 22.5/16 kg)

PARTNER WORKOUTS

Workouts are often more fun when they are done in pairs! Partner workouts bring a new dimension to the traditional CrossFit routine, adding an element of camaraderie and teamwork to the mix. They are designed for two athletes to work together to complete the workout, often sharing the workload or alternating exercises.

The workouts in this chapter are designed to push you and your partner to your limits. Each one is a testament to the adage that teamwork makes the dream work. Whether you're working on your communication, strategizing your approach, or simply trying to keep pace with your partner, these workouts will challenge you in new and exciting ways.

From AMRAPs to chippers, these partner workouts cover a broad range of exercises and formats. So grab a friend, warm up, and get ready to tackle these workouts together! It's time to prove that two is better than one.

Double Trouble AMRAP in 20 minutes

- Partner 1: 200m Run

- Partner 2: Max Double Unders

Switch when Partner 1 completes the run. Score is total number of double unders.

Jumping Jacks and Jogs AMRAP in 20 minutes:

- Buy-in: 100 Jumping Jacks (each)

  ○ Partner 1: 400m Run

  ○ Partner 2: AMRAP of 10 Push-ups and 10 Air Squats

- Cash-out: 100 Jumping Jacks (each)

Switch when Partner 1 completes the run. Repeat until 20 minutes is up.

Barbell Bonanza For time:

- 100 Thrusters (95/65 lbs - 43/30 kg)

- 100 Pull-ups

- 100 Power cleans (95/65 lbs - 43/30 kg)

- 100 Toes-to-bars

Divide the work evenly with one athlete working at a time.

Barbell Partners AMRAP in 20 minutes:

- Buy-in: 50 Synchronized Barbell Thrusters (95/65 lbs - 43/30 kg)

- ○ Partner 1: 15 Toes-to-bars

- ○ Partner 2: Hold a Plank

- Cash-out: 50 Synchronized Barbell Deadlifts (185/135 lbs - 84/61 kg)

Switch when Partner 1 completes the toes-to-bars. Hold the plank until your partner finishes their reps.

Row and Go 3 Rounds for time:

- Partner 1: Row 500 meters

- Partner 2: AMRAP of 15 Dumbbell Devil Presses (50/35 lbs - 22.5/15 kg) and 15 Box Jumps (24/20")

Switch when Partner 1 completes the row. Score is total time and rounds of AMRAP completed.

Climb the Ladder With a 30-minute running clock:

- Minute 1: 1 Burpee (each)

- Minute 2: 2 Burpees (each)

- Continue adding 1 Burpee each minute until both athletes cannot complete the required reps in the minute.
  Score is the last completed round of burpees.

Double Under Duel AMRAP in 25 minutes:

- Buy-in: 200 Double Unders (each, relay style)

  - ○ Partner 1: 15 Dumbbell Devil Presses (50/35 lbs - 22.5

/15 kg)

- ○ Partner 2: Hold a Wall Sit

- Cash-out: 200 Double Unders (each, relay style)

Switch when Partner 1 completes the devil presses. Hold the wall sit until your partner finishes their reps.

Relay Race For time:

- 400m Run

- 50 Wall Balls (20/14 lbs - 9/6 kg)

- 40 Calorie Bike

- 30 Dumbbell Snatches (50/35 lbs - 22.5/15 kg)

- 400m Run

Partner 1 completes the entire round, then Partner 2 completes the entire round. Score is total time.

Tandem Trouble AMRAP in 25 minutes

- Partner 1: 12 Kettlebell Swings (53/35 lbs - 24/16 kg)

- Partner 2: 12 Box Jumps (24/20")

- Both: 200m Run together

Partners alternate movements, both run together.

Push and Pull For time:

- 150 Push-ups

- 100 Pull-ups

- 50 Calorie Row

Split work as desired, one person works at a time.

Rowing Renegades AMRAP in 30 minutes:

- Buy-in: 2000m Row (split as desired)

  - Partner 1: 12 Burpees

  - Partner 2: Hold a Deadlift (225/155 lbs - 102/70 kg)

- Cash-out: 2000m Row (split as desired)

Switch when Partner 1 completes the burpees. Hold the deadlift until your partner finishes their reps.

Double AMRAP AMRAP in 10 minutes

- 15 Wall Balls (20/14 lbs - 9/6 kg)

- 10 Toes-to-bars
  Rest 5 minutes, then repeat.

One partner works while the other rests.

Switcheroo 4 Rounds for time:

- Partner 1: 400m Run

- Partner 2: AMRAP of 15 Dumbbell Snatches (50/35 lbs - 22.5/15 kg) and 15 Box Jumps (24/20")

Switch when Partner 1 completes the run. Repeat until both partners have completed 4 rounds.

The Long Haul For time:

- 2000m Row

- 100 Burpees

- 100 Dumbbell Devil Presses (50/35 lbs - 22.5/15 kg)

Split the work however you want, but both partners must row 1000m each.

Synchronized Swings AMRAP in 15 minutes

- 20 Synchronized Kettlebell Swings (53/35 lbs - 24/16 kg)

- 20 Synchronized Box Jumps (24/20")

Couplet Relay For time:

- Partner 1: 21-15-9 Thrusters (95/65 lbs - 43/30 kg) and Pull-ups

- Partner 2: 21-15-9 Deadlifts (225/155 lbs - 102/70 kg) and Handstand Push-ups

Partner 1 completes the first couplet, then tags Partner 2 to complete the second couplet.

See-Saw 5 Rounds for time:

- Partner 1: 500m Row

- Partner 2: Holds a Plank

Partners switch after each 500m row.

Mirror Image AMRAP in 20 minutes

- Partner 1: 15 Calorie Bike

- Partner 2: 15 Wall Balls (20/14 lbs - 9/6 kg)

- Both: 200m Run together

Partners switch movements each round, run together.

Climbing Together With a 20-minute running clock:

- Minute 1: 1 Devil Press (2x 50/35 lbs - 23/16 kg) (each)

- Minute 2: 2 Devil Press (2x 50/35 lbs - 23/16 kg) (each)

- Continue adding 1 Devil Press each minute until both athletes cannot complete the required reps in the minute.

Score is the last completed round of Devil Press.

Squat and Swing AMRAP in 25 minutes:

- Buy-in: 100 Synchronized Air Squats

  - Partner 1: 20 Kettlebell Swings (24/16 kg - 53/35 lb)

  - Partner 2: Hold a Handstand

- Cash-out: 100 Synchronized Air Squats

Switch when Partner 1 completes the kettlebell swings. Hold the handstand until your partner finishes their reps.

Push-Up Pals AMRAP in 20 minutes:

- Buy-in: 75 Synchronized Push-Ups

  - Partner 1: 15 Box Jumps (24/20")

  - Partner 2: Hold a Farmer's Carry (2x 70/53 lbs - 32/24 kg)

- Cash-out: 75 Synchronized Push-Ups

Switch when Partner 1 completes the box jumps. Hold the farmer's carry until your partner finishes their reps.

Pull-up Pairs For Time:

- Partner 1: 100 Double Unders

- Partner 2: Holds a Pull-Up Bar Hang

- Swap positions

Partner can only jump when the other partner is hanging.

Synchronized Squats AMRAP in 15 minutes:

- 30 Synchronized Wall Balls (20/14 lbs - 9/6 kg)

- 30 Synchronized Toes-to-bars

Row and Hold AMRAP in 20 minutes:

- Partner 1: Rows 500 meters

- Partner 2: Holds a Handstand

Switch after each 500 meter row.

Dumbbell Duo For Time:

- 100 Dumbbell Snatches (50/35 lbs - 22.5/15 kg), alternate every 10 reps

- 100 Synchronized Dumbbell Squats (50/35 lbs - 22.5/15 kg)

Burpee Battle AMRAP in 25 minutes:

- Partner 1: 15 Burpees

- Partner 2: Holds a Deadlift (225/155 lbs - 102/70 kg)

Switch after each set of burpees.

Box Jump Buddies For Time:

- 200 Box Jumps (24/20"), alternate every 10 reps

- While Partner 1 works, Partner 2 performs a Wall Sit

Partner Chipper For Time:

- 100 Pull-Ups

- 200 Push-Ups

- 300 Air Squats

Divide the work evenly with one athlete working at a time.

Thruster Team AMRAP in 30 minutes:

- Partner 1: 10 Thrusters (95/65 lbs - 43/30 kg)

- Partner 2: Holds a Plank

Switch after each set of thrusters.

Double Under Drill AMRAP in 20 minutes:

- Partner 1: 100 Double Unders

- Partner 2: Holds a Kettlebell in a Front Rack (2x 24/16 kg - 2x53/35 lb)

Switch after each set of double unders.

Squat and Swing Synchronization For Time:

- 200 Synchronized Kettlebell Swings (24/16 kg - 53/35 lb)

- 200 Synchronized Air Squats

BUY-IN & CASH-OUT WORKOUTS

Buy-in and cash-out workouts are an exciting twist on traditional CrossFit programming that add an extra level of intensity and strategy to your sessions. These workouts typically start (buy-in) and end (cash-out) with a set task or movement that must be completed before moving on to the main part of the workout.

The buy-in and cash-out elements can be the same or different movements and are usually designed to challenge your physical capabilities, add volume, or target specific skills. The main workout sandwiched between the buy-in and cash-out can take any form, such as an AMRAP, EMOM, or rounds for time, among others.

In this chapter, you will find a wide range of buy-in and cash-out workouts that will challenge you in new and exciting ways. Each workout has been carefully designed to provide a balanced and comprehensive training stimulus. Whether you're looking to improve your endurance, strength, speed, or skill, there's a workout here for you.

Remember, the key to these workouts is to pace yourself wisely. Don't let the excitement of the buy-in phase cause you to burn out too early, and save enough energy to complete the cash-out phase effectively. Enjoy the challenge and embrace the burn!

Death by Devils

Buy-In: 1000m Row

Then, AMRAP in 12 minutes:

- 12 Wall Balls (20/14 lbs - 9/6 kg)

- 8 Dumbbell Devil Presses (35/25 lbs - 22.5/15 kg)

Cash-Out: 100 Double Unders

Ground and Pound

Buy-In: 2 mile run

Then, 5 rounds of:

- 10 Ground-to-Overheads (95/65 lbs - 43/30 kg)

- 15 Box Jumps (24/20")

Cash-Out: 50 Burpees

Roll the Dice

Buy-In: 50/35 calorie BikeErg

Then, 4 rounds of:

- 12 Overhead Squats (115/81 lbs - 52/37 kg)

- 15 Toes-to-Bars

Cash-Out: 200m Farmer's Carry (2x 50/35 lbs - 23/16 kg)

Climb the Mountain

Buy-In: 100 Double Unders

Then, 3 rounds of:

- 5 Rope Climbs

- 10 Deadlifts (225/155 lbs - 102/70 kg)

Cash-Out: 1 mile run

Grit and Grind

Buy-In: 75 Air Squats

Then, 3 rounds of:

- 20 Kettlebell Swings (53/35 lbs - 24/16 kg)

- 20 Push-ups

Cash-Out: 75 Air Squats

Metcon Madness

Buy-In: 30 Calorie Row

Then, 2 rounds of:

- 10 Muscle-ups

- 20 Dumbbell Snatches (50/35 lbs - 23/16 kg)

Cash-Out: 30 Calorie Row

Press On

Buy-In: 50 Push Presses (95/65 lbs - 43/30 kg)

Then, AMRAP in 15 minutes:

- 5 Pull-ups

- 10 Push-ups

- 15 Air Squats

Cash-Out: 50 Push Presses (95/65 lbs - 43/30 kg)

Calorie Crusher

Buy-In: 40/30 Calorie Assault Bike

Then, 5 rounds of:

- 10 Overhead Squats (135/96 lbs - 61/43 kg)

- 15 Box Jump Overs (24/20")

Cash-Out: 40/30 Calorie Assault Bike

Sprint and Swing

Buy-In: 400m Sprint

Then, 4 rounds of:

- 20 Kettlebell Swings (53/35 lbs - 24/16 kg)

- 40 Double Unders

Cash-Out: 400m Sprint

Barbell Brigade

Buy-In: 50 Deadlifts (135/95 lbs)

Then, 3 rounds of:

- 15 Thrusters (95/65 lbs)

- 15 Chest-to-Bar Pull-ups

Cash-Out: 50 Deadlifts (135/96 lbs - 61/43 kg)

Iron Will

Buy-In: 2 rounds of

- 25 Calorie Row

- 25 Air Squats

Then, 3 rounds of:

- 10 Deadlifts (225/155 lbs - 102/70 kg)

- 15 Toes-to-Bars

- 20 Box Jumps (24/20")

Cash-Out: 2 rounds of

- 25 Calorie Row

- 25 Air Squats

True Grit

Buy-In: 50 Wall Balls (20/14 lbs - 9/6 kg)

Then, 4 rounds of:

- 12 Dumbbell Snatches (50/35 lbs - 23/16 kg)

- 15 Pull-ups

- 18 Kettlebell Swings (50/35 lbs - 23/16 kg)

Cash-Out: 50 Wall Balls (20/14 lbs - 9/6 kg)

Mountain Mover

Buy-In: 3 rounds of

- 10 Calorie BikeErg

- 10 Push-ups

Then, 5 rounds of:

- 8 Overhead Squats (115/81 lbs - 52/37 kg)

- 12 Chest-to-Bar Pull-ups

- 16 Double Unders

Cash-Out: 3 rounds of

- 10 Calorie BikeErg

- 10 Push-ups

Momentum Shift

Buy-In: 1000m Row

Then, 5 rounds of:

- 5 Clean and Jerks (135/95 lbs - 61/43 kg)

- 10 Burpee Box Jumps (24/20 in)

- 15 GHD Sit-ups

Cash-Out: 1000m Row

Resolve Booster

Buy-In: 50 Dumbbell Devil Presses (2x 50/35 lbs - 23/16 kg)

Then, 3 rounds of:

- 20 Wall Balls (20/14 lbs; 9/6 kg)

- 30 Double Unders

- 40 Air Squats

Cash-Out: 50 Dumbbell Devil Presses (2x 50/35 lbs - 23/16 kg)

Steel Spirit

Buy-In: 3 rounds of

- 15 Calorie BikeErg

- 15 Kettlebell Swings (53/35 lbs - 24/16 kg)

Then, 4 rounds of:

- 10 Front Squats (155/105 lbs - 70/47.5 kg)

- 15 Toes-to-Bars

- 20 Double Unders

Cash-Out: 3 rounds of

- 15 Calorie BikeErg

- 15 Kettlebell Swings (53/35 lbs - 24/16 kg)

Grit and Grind

Buy-In: 2 rounds of

- 20 Calorie Row

- 20 Push-ups

Then, 3 rounds of:

- 12 Deadlifts (225/155 lbs - 102/70 kg)

- 18 Pull-ups

- 24 Box Jumps (24/20")

Cash-Out: 2 rounds of

- 20 Calorie Row

- 20 Push-ups

Heart Charger

Buy-In: 3 rounds of

- 10 Calorie SkiErg

- 10 Air Squats

Then, 5 rounds of:

- 5 Power Cleans (185/125 lbs - 84/57 kg)

- 10 Chest-to-Bar Pull-ups

- 15 Double Unders

Cash-Out: 3 rounds of

- 10 Calorie SkiErg

- 10 Air Squats

Resilience Raiser

Buy-In: 4 rounds of

- 15 Calorie BikeErg

- 15 Kettlebell Swings (53/35 lbs - 24/16 kg)

Then, 4 rounds of:

- 8 Front Squats (155/105 lbs - 70/47.5 kg)

- 12 Toes-to-Bars

- 16 Double Unders

Cash-Out: 4 rounds of

- 15 Calorie BikeErg

- 15 Kettlebell Swings (53/35 lbs - 24/16 kg)

Rapid Recharge

Buy-In: 100 Double Unders

Then, 4 rounds of:

- 10 Clean and Jerks (135/95 lbs - 61/43 kg)

- 15 Burpee Box Jumps (24/20")

- 20 GHD Sit-ups

Cash-Out: 100 Double Unders

Strength Surge

Buy-In: 50 Dumbbell Devil Presses (2x 50/35 lbs - 23/16 kg)

Then, 4 rounds of:

- 15 Wall Balls (20/14 lbs; 9/6 kg)

- 25 Double Unders

- 35 Air Squats

Cash-Out: 50 Dumbbell Devil Presses (2x 50/35 lbs - 23/16 kg)

Tenacity Tester

Buy-In: 3 rounds of

- 10 Calorie Row

- 10 Air Squats

Then, 5 rounds of:

- 7 Overhead Squats (115/80 lbs - 52/36 kg)

- 14 Chest-to-Bar Pull-ups

- 21 Double Unders

Cash-Out: 3 rounds of

- 10 Calorie Row

- 10 Air Squats

Willpower Warrior

Buy-In: 2 rounds of

- 15 Calorie SkiErg

- 15 Kettlebell Swings (53/35 lbs - 24/16 kg)

Then, 4 rounds of:

- 12 Front Squats (155/105 lbs - 70/47.5 kg)

- 16 Toes-to-Bars

- 20 Double Unders

Cash-Out: 2 rounds of

- 15 Calorie SkiErg

- 15 Kettlebell Swings (53/35 lbs - 24/16 kg)

MOBILITY AND FLEXIBILITY WORKOUTS

Mobility and flexibility are often underemphasized in many training programs, yet they are critical aspects of overall fitness and health. While mobility refers to the ability of a joint to move through its full range of motion, flexibility pertains to the length and stretchability of the muscles. Optimal performance, injury prevention, and improved recovery are just a few benefits gained from incorporating regular mobility and flexibility exercises into your routine.

In this chapter, we'll provide a variety of workouts designed specifically to improve your mobility and flexibility. These workouts will incorporate dynamic movements, static stretches, yoga poses, and bodyweight exercises designed to increase joint mobility, improve muscle flexibility, and promote better movement quality.

Whether you're an elite athlete looking to enhance performance, or someone seeking to maintain functional fitness and ease of movement in everyday life, these workouts will offer valuable additions to your training regimen. The goal is not just to become stronger, faster, or more enduring, but also to move with greater ease and grace. So, let's get mobile and flexible!

Deep Stretch Session

1. 2-minute Forward Fold

2. 2-minute Low Lunge (each side)

3. 2-minute Pigeon Pose (each side)

4. 2-minute Butterfly Stretch

5. 2-minute Seated Forward Bend

6. 1-minute Child's Pose

7. 1-minute Upward Dog

Notes: Hold each pose for the stated duration, focusing on deep, controlled breathing. Try to relax into each pose and deepen the stretch as you exhale.

Full Body Mobility Flow

1. 10 Cat-Cow Stretches

2. 10 Shoulder Rolls (each direction)

3. 10 Hip Circles (each direction)

4. 10 Knee Circles (each direction)

5. 10 Ankle Rolls (each direction)

6. 5 Sun Salutations

7. 10 Spinal Rotations (each side)

Notes: Complete the movements in a slow and controlled manner, focusing on the full range of motion. This workout is not about speed but about improving your mobility.

Yoga for Athletes

1. 2-minute Downward Dog

2. 1-minute Warrior I (each side)

3. 1-minute Warrior II (each side)

4. 1-minute Triangle Pose (each side)

5. 2-minute Seated Twist (each side)

6. 2-minute Bridge Pose

7. 2-minute Legs-Up-The-Wall Pose

Notes: Hold each pose for the stated duration, focusing on deep, controlled breathing. Each pose is designed to target different muscle groups and improve flexibility.

Hip Mobility Magic

1. 10 Lizard Pose (each side)

2. 10 Pigeon Pose (each side)

3. 10 Butterfly Stretches

4. 10 Seated Leg Cradle (each side)

5. 10 Frog Pose

6. 10 Kneeling Hip Flexor Stretch (each side)

Notes: Complete the movements in a slow and controlled manner, focusing on the full range of motion. This workout specifically targets the hips, aiming to improve mobility and flexibility.

Upper Body Opener

1. 2-minute Doorway Stretch (each side)

2. 2-minute Thread the Needle Pose (each side)

3. 2-minute Eagle Arm Stretch (each side)

4. 1-minute Neck Rolls (each direction)

5. 2-minute Extended Puppy Pose

6. 1-minute Wrist Stretch (each direction)

Notes: This sequence is designed to stretch and open up the upper body, including the shoulders, chest, neck, and wrists. Hold each pose for the stated duration, focusing on deep, controlled breathing.

Shoulder Release Routine

1. 10 Arm Circles (each direction)

2. 10 Across the Chest Arm Stretches (each side)

3. 2-minute Doorway Stretch (each side)

4. 1-minute Thread the Needle Pose (each side)

5. 10 Shoulder Rolls (each direction)

6. 2-minute Eagle Arm Stretch (each side)

Notes: This sequence is designed to specifically target the shoulders, helping to release tension and improve flexibility after a heavy upper body workout.

Hip and Hamstring Harmony

1. 2-minute Forward Fold

2. 2-minute Low Lunge (each side)

3. 2-minute Pigeon Pose (each side)

4. 2-minute Seated Forward Bend

5. 2-minute Butterfly Stretch

6. 2-minute Lizard Pose (each side)

Notes: This routine focuses on the hips and hamstrings, perfect for post-lower body workout or to improve overall flexibility in these areas.

Chest and Tricep Tranquility

1. 2-minute Doorway Stretch (each side)

2. 2-minute Upward Dog

3. 1-minute Extended Puppy Pose

4. 2-minute Sphinx Pose

    5. 2-minute Lying Chest Stretch (each side)

    6. 2-minute Overhead Tricep Stretch (each side)

Notes: A sequence designed to open up the chest and stretch out the triceps. Ideal for post-workout recovery after any pressing movements.

Back and Lat Loosener

    1. 2-minute Child's Pose with Extended Arms

    2. 1-minute Cat-Cow Stretches

    3. 2-minute Sphinx Pose

    4. 2-minute Seated Forward Bend

    5. 2-minute Downward Dog

    6. 2-minute Thread the Needle Pose (each side)

Notes: This sequence focuses on stretching the muscles of the back and lats, perfect for post-pull up or rowing sessions.

Quad and Calf Calm

    1. 2-minute Low Lunge (each side)

    2. 2-minute Pigeon Pose with Quad Stretch (each side)

    3. 2-minute Standing Quad Stretch (each side)

    4. 2-minute Downward Dog

    5. 2-minute Standing Calf Stretch (each side)

6. 2-minute Seated Forward Bend

Notes: A post-workout sequence designed to target the quads and calves, perfect for recovery after squats, running, or biking.

SCALING OPTIONS

When it comes to CrossFit and functional fitness, one of the key principles is scalability. Scalability ensures that every individual, regardless of their current fitness level or ability, can participate in workouts and make progress towards their goals. This chapter will provide an overview of scaling options, techniques, and examples to help you better understand how to modify workouts and movements to meet your individual needs and abilities.

Reducing the Load

One of the simplest ways to scale a workout is to reduce the load or weight used for a given movement. This can be particularly helpful for beginners or those recovering from an injury. Choose a weight that allows you to maintain proper form and technique while still providing a challenging workout.

Example: If a workout prescribes 135 lbs/60 kg for a barbell movement, you can scale it down to 95 lbs/43 kg or even lower, depending on your abilities and comfort level.

Reducing Repetitions

Another effective way to scale a workout is by reducing the number of repetitions or rounds. This can help maintain the intended stimulus of the workout while making it more manageable for those who are less experienced or have limited endurance.

Example: If a workout calls for 5 rounds of 20 reps, you can scale it down to 3 rounds of 15 reps or even lower, depending on your current fitness level.

Modifying Movements

Modifying or substituting movements can be an effective way to scale a workout, especially when a particular movement is challenging due to mobility, strength, or skill limitations. It's important to choose a similar movement that still targets the same muscle groups and provides a comparable workout stimulus.

Example: If a workout includes muscle-ups, you can scale them to pull-ups and dips or even ring rows and push-ups, depending on your abilities.

Adjusting Time Caps and Rest Periods

Altering the time cap or adding rest periods can also help scale a workout to your fitness level. A longer time cap provides more time to complete the workout, while shorter rest periods can make the workout more intense.

Example: If a workout has a 15-minute time cap, you can scale it to a 20-minute cap, allowing you more time to complete the movements. Alternatively, if a workout includes 1-minute rest between rounds, you can scale it to 2 minutes of rest to allow for more recovery time.

Using Assistance or Support

Utilizing assistance or support can make certain movements more accessible. For example, using a band for pull-ups or push-ups, or using a box for assisted dips or pistols.

Example: If a workout includes strict handstand push-ups, you can scale them by using a box for piked handstand push-ups, or by performing regular push-ups with your feet elevated on a box.

Remember, scaling is not a sign of weakness or failure. It's a tool that allows you to make progress at your own pace and ensures that you're working out safely and effectively. Always consult with a coach or experienced athlete if you're unsure of how to scale a workout or movement to meet your needs. Ultimately, the goal is to challenge yourself, improve your fitness, and enjoy the process.

NUTRITION AND RECOVERY

Cross Training & CrossFit is not just about the workouts; it's also about promoting a holistic approach to health, which includes proper nutrition and recovery. These two factors are crucial for enhancing performance, promoting muscle growth and repair, and preventing injury.

Nutrition

In Cross Training & CrossFit, nutrition is viewed as the foundation of health and fitness. Without proper nutrition, your body won't have the fuel it needs to perform at its best, and your progress may be hindered. Here's a basic guide to nutrition for CrossFit:

1. **Macronutrients**: Make sure your diet is well-balanced and includes adequate amounts of protein (for muscle repair and growth), carbohydrates (for energy), and fats (for energy and various bodily functions).

2. **Micronutrients**: Vitamins and minerals are also essential

for your body's processes, including energy production, bone health, and immune function.

3. **Hydration**: Water is vital for various bodily functions, including digestion and temperature regulation. Make sure you're drinking enough water each day, especially around workouts.

4. **Timing**: When you eat is also important. Try to have a balanced meal 2-3 hours before your workout and a protein-rich snack or meal afterward to help with recovery.

5. **Quality**: Aim for whole, unprocessed foods whenever possible. They're more nutrient-dense and generally healthier than highly processed foods.

Recovery

Recovery is the time when your body repairs and strengthens itself in the time between workouts. It's one of the most important aspects of fitness, and neglecting it can lead to overtraining, injuries, and plateaus. Here are some recovery methods to incorporate into your routine:

1. **Rest**: Make sure you're getting enough sleep each night. Sleep is when a lot of your body's recovery processes occur.

2. **Active Recovery**: Light activities on your rest days, like walking or yoga, can help improve blood flow and speed up the recovery process.

3. **Mobility Work**: Regular stretching and mobility work can

help maintain a full range of motion and prevent injuries.

4. **Hydration and Nutrition**: As mentioned above, staying hydrated and eating a well-balanced diet can support recovery.

5. **Mental Recovery**: Practices like meditation and mindfulness can help manage stress, which can, in turn, improve physical recovery.

Remember, everyone is different, so it may take some time and experimentation to find what works best for you in terms of nutrition and recovery. It's always a good idea to consult with a healthcare professional or a registered dietitian if you're unsure or if you have specific dietary needs.

PROGRAMMING

When it comes to CrossFit/Cross Training, programming is an integral part of achieving success. It's not just about working out with high intensity, but about carefully planning and balancing different types of workouts and movements over time. Proper programming ensures athletes progress, avoid injuries, and maintain enthusiasm for the long term.

Programming in CrossFit/Cross Training can be complex due to the sheer variety of exercises, workout styles, and goals of the program. It can include strength training, metabolic conditioning, mobility work, skill-based training, and much more. The key is to find the right balance and progression for each individual or group of athletes.

Considerations for Effective Programming

Here are some important considerations for effective CrossFit/Cross Training programming:

- **Goal Setting:** Understand what you or your athletes want to achieve. Whether it's improving overall fitness, gaining strength, increasing endurance, or preparing for a competition, your programming should align with these goals.

- **Variety and Balance:** CrossFit/Cross Training is all about variety, but this needs to be balanced. Ensure you're not neglecting any areas such as strength, endurance, flexibility, or skill work.

- **Progression:** Workouts should progressively challenge athletes, increasing in intensity, complexity, or volume over time to drive continual adaptation and prevent plateaus.

- **Recovery:** Rest and recovery are just as important as the workouts themselves. Make sure to incorporate rest days and lighter recovery workouts into your programming.

- **Scalability:** Not all athletes will be at the same level. Workouts should be scalable to accommodate different levels of fitness and skill.

- **Consistency:** While variety is important, so is consistency. Repeating certain workouts or types of workouts allows athletes to see their progress over time.

Creating a Weekly CrossFit/Cross Training Program

While there's no one-size-fits-all approach, here's an example of how you might structure a week of CrossFit/Cross Training:

- **Monday:** Strength focus (e.g., squats, deadlifts, presses)

- **Tuesday:** Metabolic conditioning (e.g., AMRAP, ladder workouts)

- **Wednesday:** Skill work and mobility (e.g., gymnastics movements, mobility exercises)

- **Thursday:** Active recovery (e.g., light cardio, stretching)

- **Friday:** Mixed modal (e.g., combination of strength and metabolic conditioning)

- **Saturday:** Endurance or longer workout

- **Sunday:** Rest

Remember, this is just an example. The actual program should be tailored to the individual or group, considering their goals, abilities, and schedule.

Effective programming is both a science and an art. It requires understanding the principles of fitness and training, but also knowing your athletes and being able to adapt and be creative. With thoughtful and balanced programming, you can help ensure that every Cross-Fit/Cross Training workout brings you one step closer to your fitness goals.

CONCLUSION AND NEXT STEPS

In this book, we've taken a deep dive into the exciting and challenging world of CrossFit/Cross Training. From understanding the fundamentals of this fitness discipline to exploring various workouts and training strategies, we hope you've found the information helpful and inspiring.

CrossFit/Cross Training is not just about physical strength or endurance; it's about forging a strong mind-body connection, embracing challenges, and continually striving for progress—not perfection. It's about the community you build, the personal barriers you break, and the joy of achieving goals you once thought were out of reach.

Remember, everyone's CrossFit/Cross Training journey is unique. Don't compare your progress with others. Instead, focus on your personal growth, both physically and mentally. Listen to your body, scale when necessary, and push yourself when you feel ready.

Next Steps

What comes next in your CrossFit/Cross Training journey is entirely up to you, but here are a few suggestions:

Apply what you've learned: Use the workouts and strategies in this book to enhance your own training or the programming at your gym. Remember, the key is variety and balance.

Keep Learning: The world of CrossFit/Cross Training is always evolving. Stay updated with the latest training techniques, workout ideas, and scientific research. Attend seminars, connect with the CrossFit/Cross Training community, and don't hesitate to learn from others.

Take Care of Your Body: Remember, recovery and nutrition are as important as your workouts. Prioritize sleep, eat a balanced diet, and listen to your body's signals. Consider working with a nutritionist or physiotherapist to further optimize your performance and recovery.

Compete: If you're feeling adventurous and want to test your skills, consider participating in a CrossFit/Cross Training competition. It can be a local event or even the CrossFit Games if you're up for the challenge. Competing can be a great way to benchmark your progress and meet other passionate athletes.

Share the Knowledge: If you're an experienced CrossFit/Cross Training athlete or a coach, consider helping others in their fitness journey. Share your knowledge, mentor new athletes, or even write about your experiences.

No matter what your next steps look like, remember why you started. Keep that passion alive, and let it fuel your journey.

Thank you for embarking on this CrossFit/Cross Training journey with us. Here's to many more workouts, personal records, and moments of triumph ahead. Keep moving, stay strong, and never stop believing in your potential.

Good luck, and see you at the box!

Printed in Great Britain
by Amazon